Drug Treatment of the Rheumatic Diseases

Drug Treatment of the Rheumatic Diseases

Edited by
F. Dudley Hart

MTP PRESS LIMITED *International Medical Publishers*

Drug Treatment of the Rheumatic Diseases

Published in UK, Europe and Middle East
by MTP Press Limited
Falcon House
Lancaster
England

Second Printing
ISBN 0-85200-506-7

MTP PRESS LIMITED International Medical Publishers

Printed at Bright Sun Printing Press Co. Ltd., Hong Kong

Preface

When I qualified in medicine in Edinburgh and was doing my intern posts in 1934-5, there was, outside Spas and so-called Health Centres, not only little interest shown in the rheumatic disorders but also very few drugs available with which to treat them. For the treatment of gout we had colchicine, for the treatment of rheumatoid arthritis gold salts and aspirin. As no drugs greatly helped patients with ankylosing spondylitis radiotherapy was considered the best therapy available. Phenacetin and amidopyrine, useful agents at the time, later became supplanted and replaced, but compound codeine tablets held their place in popularity. The advent of the sulphonamide drugs and antibiotics between 1935 and 1944 changed the face of medicine as regards the effective treatment of many infective and postinfective disorders and rheumatic fever became a rare disorder in Europe. Later, between 1946 and 1950 we saw tuberculous disease controlled and largely conquered.

At this time, drug treatment of the rheumatic disorders appeared to be lagging behind, but in 1949 Philip Hench and his colleagues at the Mayo Clinic dramatically demonstrated the effects of cortisone in rheumatoid arthritis and in other disorders. This revolutionised rheumatology. The fact that something really worked in these disorders acted like a shot in the arm to a rather tired and sluggish speciality. The Cinderella of Medicine, almost overnight, became respectable and rather fashionable and attractive to specialists in many fields, and many workers from different disciplines entered the field of rheumatism research with quite dramatic results.

On the pharmacological front, exciting things started to happen. Phenylbutazone appeared in 1952 and rapidly proved to be a truly effective analgesic-anti-inflammatory-antipyretic agent, and in the same year, probenecid became available as the first practical useful uricosuric agent. Since then, many new drugs have appeared and instead of the poor bewildered general practitioner having difficulty in finding a suitable agent for a particular patient his bewilderment lies now in deciding which of the many agents available he should use.

This book is aimed at helping that bewildered clinician. We hope that its contents prove useful to him. Part I is a brief outline of the pharmacological properties, actions, indications and contra-indications and drug interactions of the drugs in current use in rheumatology, while Part II discusses the practical treatment of the more common rheumatic and arthritic disorders. But it is a sobering and somewhat depressing thought that although there are more therapeutic agents available today than were ever known to our predecessors, it is likely that more traditional, herbal, homeopathic and homely agents are being purchased across the country than are being obtained on prescription, and are being swallowed to relieve symptoms of conditions we should all be controlling or curing. We still await the perfect analgesic and anti-inflammatory drug, effective, cheap, non-toxic, but the therapeutic advances in rheumatology in my time have, nevertheless, been quite extraordinary.

I must, as editor, thank all contributors to this book for their excellent co-operation, the publishers, and Graeme Avery in particular, for their ever-ready help and efficiency on all occasions, to Brian Lacey, Professor of Bacteriology at Westminster Hospital, London, for his advice regarding antibiotic therapy, and to Mrs Valerie Mayblatt and Miss Linda Terrett for their highly efficient and invaluable secretarial assistance.

F. Dudley Hart
London, January 1978

Contributors

Ansell, Barbara, M.
Clinical Research Centre, Northwick Park Hospital, Watford Road, Harrow, Middlesex HA1 3UJ, England.

Christian, Charles, L.
The Hospital for Special Surgery, Rheumatic Diseases Unit, 535 E 70th Street, New York, NY 10021, USA.

Emmerson, Bryan, T.
Professor of Medicine, University of Queensland, Princess Alexandra Hospital, Brisbane, Australia 4102, Australia.

Gratwick, Geoffrey
Post Doctoral Fellow, Hospital for Special Surgery, Cornell University, 535 E 70th Street, New York, NY 10021, USA.

Hart, F. Dudley
Consulting Physician, Westminster Hospital; Physician, Hospital of St. John and St. Elizabeth, London, England.

Huskisson, Edward, C.
Senior Lecturer, Department of Rheumatology, St. Bartholomew's Hospital, London EC1A 7BE, England.

Kagen, Lawrence
The Hospital for Special Surgery, Rheumatic Diseases Unit, 535 E 70th Street, New York, NY 10021, USA.

Contents

Part II: Therapeutics

Chapter I

General Principles

No group of disorders causes so much persistent pain and so much prolonged illness and distress as do the rheumatic diseases, and few patients need so many drugs so regularly for what has rightly been called the 'long pain'.

1. The Nature of Rheumatic Pain

Pain in the rheumatic sufferer is a diabolical cocktail (fig. 1) with many ingredients: local pain, general aching and 'unwellness', fever, local and general weakness, depression, anxiety, increased fatiguability, systemic manifestations, and, on top of all these, unpleasant drug reactions and interactions in many cases. Some of these ingredients come through at conscious clinical level ('My wrists ache, Doctor, and my feet are painful so I can hardly walk.') Others, like nausea, weakness and increased fatiguability, are so much a part of the patient's life that they cease to be complaints and are taken for granted: it is only when they are removed as with a truly effective treatment or in natural remission, that the patient suddenly notices the glorious difference.

Long pains and long illnesses are soul destroying, sapping the morale of even the most stoical and uncomplaining patient, and no diseases last quite so long and break up lives quite so much as the rheumatic disorders. It is the chronic nature of these diseases and the long-term programme of drug administration that sets the rheumatic disorders apart from most others. Non-compliance, the failure to take their prescribed medicines, is less of a problem with rheumatic sufferers than, let us say, the hypertensive or the hyperlipoproteinaemic patient, because if the rheumatic patient doesn't take medication the pains rapidly return. Non-compliance in arthritic sufferers often means either that the drug isn't very effective or it is toxic and upsetting the patient, and in both cases the physician should take heed and act accordingly.

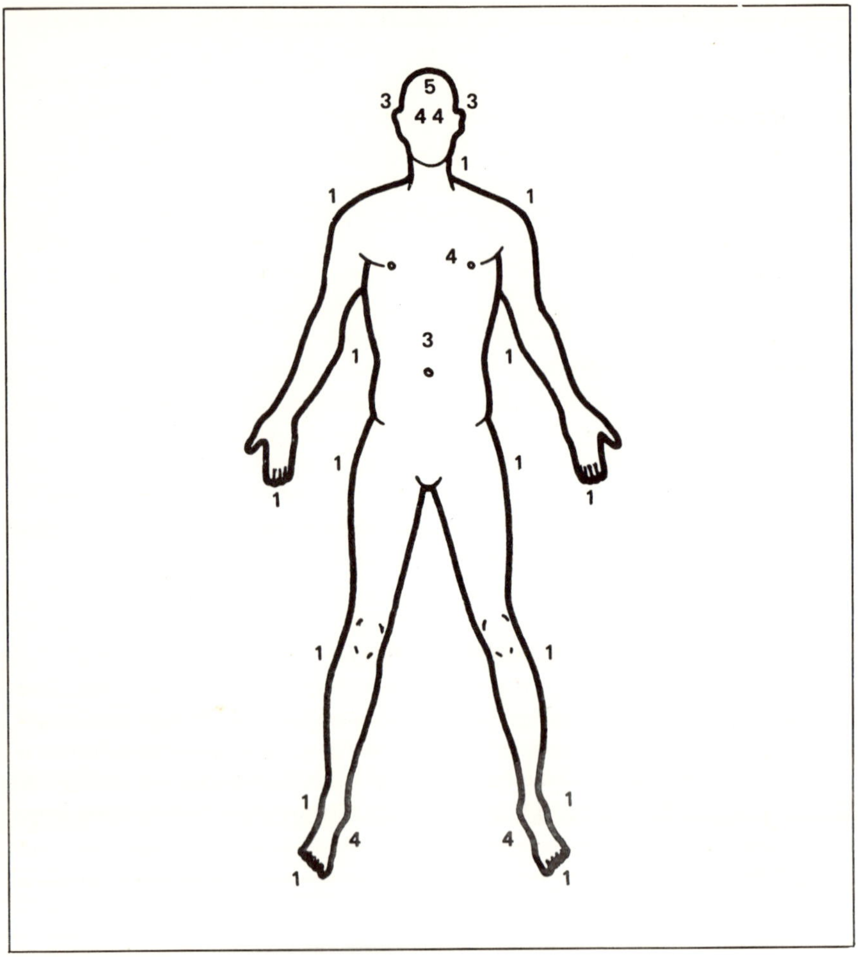

Fig. 1. The pain cocktail of rheumatoid disease.

1. Peripheral joint pain, swelling, stiffness and weakness.
2. Systemic illness — fever, anaemia, anorexia etc.
3. Iatrogenic overtones — dyspepsia, diarrhoea, nausea, tinnitus etc.
4. Extra-articular manifestations — neuropathy, pericarditis, episcleritis, scleritis, ulcerative nodules over pressure points, keratoconjunctivitis etc.
5. Psychic overtones — depression, anxiety, tension.

Calling for:

1. Anti-inflammatory and analgesic agents and physical methods.
2. Iron, perhaps folic acid, vitamins, nursing, blood transfusions if anaemia severe from several factors.
3. Drug control and change of drugs.
4. Appropriate symptomatic therapy.
5. Antidepresssants, antianxiety drugs, personal communication, occupation.

For this reason there must be complete harmony (rapport) between physician and patient, with no secrets either way.

For this, one physician one patient is the ideal. It is impossible for a new physician to appreciate the clinical, social, psychological and pharmacological 'niceties' of a patient seen for the first time with notes 4cm thick and a history going back 10 years — the patient loses confidence in the process and often much more. The most difficult patient to treat is the one who has lost all confidence in the management of her case, in her physician, in her physiotherapist and in her drugs. It is a characteristic of depression that negatives increase: no energy, no appetite, no sex desire, and sometimes no response to drugs which previously helped.

This book is devoted entirely to the drug treatment of the different rheumatic disorders. Drugs are used to reduce and control pain and inflammation and its attendant swelling, stiffness and weakness in articular and periarticular structures; to produce better use of the joints with less discomfort and a greater range of activities within the total therapeutic programme; to help combat depression and anxiety; and to make nights less painful and more restful — in a word, to make life more livable. In a few rare cases, drug therapy aims at correcting a metabolic defect or actually reversing (curing) a disease process. Drugs may also help correct secondary deficiencies in vitamins, hormones, minerals and other substances, and although no attempt is made in this book to touch on surgical, physical or occupational therapy, drugs do play their part in making these other therapies more efficient and less painful.

Prescriptions are important in rheumatology but so is the prescriber. The rheumatic patient, like the diabetic, should know what the medicine she takes is supposed to do and what toxic effects it may have. She is her own dispenser in her own home for most of the time and should have very clear ideas of what to expect of her therapy. It is extraordinary even today how many arthritic patients are in blind ignorance of what drugs they are taking. The rapport between patient and her physician should extend to her applied therapeutics: this has a two way educational effect on both.

One final point must be strongly emphasised, and that is that drug therapy is merely a part of the treatment and management of the arthritic sufferer. Often of equal importance are physical and surgical measures, and what might be called psychological support. This book is devoted only to drug therapy, but the reader must understand that, though very important, this is not by any means the only or even the major part of treatment in this group of disorders.

2. Classification of Antirheumatic Drugs

Classification is an essential prelude to rational use of antirheumatic drugs and is increasingly important with the increasing number of drugs available. The different classes of antirheumatic drugs are shown in table I.

Table I. Classification of antirheumatic drugs

1. *Non-Specific or Symptomatic Remedies*
   a) Simple analgesics — e.g. paracetamol (acetaminophen)
   b) Analgesics with minor anti-inflammatory properties — e.g. propionic acid derivatives such as ibuprofen and similar compounds
   c) Analgesics with major anti-inflammatory properties — e.g. aspirin, indomethacin and phenylbutazone
   d) Pure non-analgesic anti-inflammatory drugs — corticosteroids

2. *Specific Drugs for Particular Diseases*
   a) Rheumatoid arthritis — e.g. gold, penicillamine
   b) Gout — e.g. colchicine, allopurinol, probenecid, benzbromarone

A distinction must first be made between non-specific or symptomatic remedies and those which are specific to particular diseases. Non-specific remedies relieve symptoms regardless of the nature of the disease and do not alter the course or outcome of the disease. The action of specific remedies is dependent on the underlying disease process, the course and outcome of which may be altered.

2.1 Simple Analgesics

Simple analgesics, like paracetamol (acetaminophen), relieve pain without having any anti-inflammatory action. They act within 30 to 60 minutes and their effect lasts for about 4 to 6 hours. A second dose reproduces the effect of the first, so that in most cases there is little point in giving regular dosage. They are used when required for pain which is intermittent and are not particularly effective in inflammatory disorders.

2.2 Non-Steroidal Anti-Inflammatory Analgesics

There are two different types of non-steroidal anti-inflammatory analgesic drugs. The traditional type, including aspirin, indomethacin and phenylbutazone, have major anti-inflammatory effects but commonly produce gastric and other side-effects. The newer drugs, such as propionic acid derivatives like ibuprofen, have less anti-inflammatory effect but much less tendency to cause side-effects. They are less suitable for diseases in which inflammation is prominent and more suitable for non-inflammatory conditions.

In the absence of inflammation, the use of drugs like phenylbutazone is in most cases unnecessary and the risks may be considered unjustifiable. Both these types of drug have analgesic properties and are effective in any painful condition; the more active, more recently introduced anti-inflammatory drugs like naproxen and fenoprofen are as effective as high dose aspirin in relieving symptoms and these two groups may be regarded as a spectrum of potency rather than as distinct entities.

2.3 Corticosteroids

Corticosteroids relieve pain only by their anti-inflammatory action. Though they represent the most effective anti-inflammatory drugs available, there is no evidence that they alter the outcome of rheumatoid arthritis and in doses required to control it, they produce features of Cushing's disease. Local corticosteroids are useful in many conditions.

The anti-inflammatory groups of drugs are arranged in increasing order of both effectiveness and toxicity. Use of the safest and best tolerated drug first is the most satisfactory philosophy for choosing antirheumatic drugs.

2.4 Drugs with a Specific Action

The most potent drugs for rheumatoid arthritis and, again, the most toxic are those which have a 'specific' action. These drugs act slowly, taking 4 to 6 months to achieve their maximum effect. Their action on joints is accompanied by effects on extra-articular features of the disease and on erythrocyte sedimentation rate (ESR) and rheumatoid factor titre. Some of these compounds are capable of altering the outcome of the disease, as judged by progression of radiological changes.

There are a number of drugs which have a similar specific type of action in other rheumatic diseases, such as allopurinol for gout and antibiotics for septic arthritis.

2.5 Drugs to Improve General Well-Being

There are also many other classes of drugs which may be required for patients with arthritis, including antidepressants, antianxiety drugs, hypnotics, iron and vitamins.

3. A Rational Basis for Symptomatic Therapy

It is essential to have some plan for choosing antirheumatic drugs. The drug treatment plan has two objects.

1) It is directed at finding for each patient the drug which combines greatest effectiveness and least toxicity. There is marked between-patient variability in response to anti-inflammatory drugs — *differences between patients are greater than differences between drugs,* so that it is often necessary to try a number of compounds before finding the best for a particular patient.

2) It is designed to avoid using the more toxic drugs in patients who don't really need them and in patients who could be treated just as well with safer drugs.

The following scheme is based on the principle of using the safest and best tolerated drugs first. It is suitable as a guide to symptomatic therapy in a wide variety of rheumatic diseases such as rheumatoid arthritis, osteoarthrosis, soft tissue rheumatism and back pain. Some exceptions are mentioned below.

a) **Step 1:** In patients with mild or intermittent pain, use simple analgesics, taken on demand.

b) **Step 2:** If regular treatment is required, start with a propionic acid derivative such as naproxen or fenoprofen. Prescribe a drug for 2 weeks then review progress. If one drug is not effective or causes side-effects, try another. Consider at this stage non-steroidal anti-inflammatory drugs with properties like propionic acid derivatives, such as tolmetin or azapropazone.

c) **Step 3:** Consider supplementing regular anti-inflammatory therapy with indomethacin at night for the relief of morning stiffness, pain at night and sleep disturbance, or with simple analgesics taken on demand when pain is not relieved. Take one step at a time and review and record the results so that patients do not accumulate a supply of drugs which is not helpful.

d) **Step 4:** In patients with active inflammatory disease, who have failed to respond to propionic acid derivatives, move on to the major anti-inflammatory group, aspirin, indomethacin and phenylbutazone. *Systemic corticosteroids have no place in such a scheme.* They should be reserved for specific indications such as polymyalgia rheumatica or polymyositis.

e) **Step 5:** Specific therapy follows on as the next step. In patients with rheumatoid arthritis for example, penicillamine or gold salts should be used for a patient who has been through the non-steroidal anti-inflammatory drug routine but still has persistent active disease.

It is the safety first philosophy which has, in the opinion of many clinicians, displaced aspirin as the first line of symptomatic treatment of diseases like rheumatoid arthritis. The more active propionic acid derivatives such as naproxen and fenoprofen are as effective as full doses of aspirin but with a striking reduction in the incidence of side-effects and a substantial increase in the number of patients able to continue with the treatment. Aspirin may still be preferred in patients with very active inflammatory rheumatoid arthritis and for patients who cannot afford the newer and more expensive drugs. Some patients undoubtedly like aspirin and do well on it. Slow release, enteric coated or other 'special' aspirin preparations may help but their cost rises with their formulation 'sophistication' and evidence for their advantages is in many instances unconvincing. Some clinicians continue to prefer aspirin as the first line of treatment; *the end point is the same whatever the scheme — the right drug for each individual patient.*

A scheme of this type has no place in the management of acute gout (see chapter X), when the course of treatment is short enough to avoid side-effects and the most potent anti-inflammatory drugs can be used initially. The plan will, however, need to be varied according to the patient's previous therapeutic experiences and response. In children, many of the newer drugs have not been adequately tested and aspirin remains the first choice. The above scheme should nevertheless prove satisfactory for most adult patients.

Reference and Recommended Reading

Huskisson, E.C.: Reports on Rheumatic Diseases, No. 54 (Arthritis and Rheumatism Council, London 1974).

Chapter II

Non-Steroidal Anti-inflammatory Analgesics

The non-steroidal anti-inflammatory analgesics (NSAID'S) do not cure or permanently reverse the inflammatory process in any arthropathy, but by reducing swelling and pain and allowing better joint function, do help the clinical condition considerably. By suppressing the inflammatory process in a chronic disease like rheumatoid arthritis life is made easier and where natural remission occurs in a short time, as in gout, the time off work and period of incapacity is reduced to a minimum. With all their drawbacks and toxic potentialities, the non-steroidal anti-inflammatory analgesics remain necessary for and beneficial to most sufferers with rheumatic complaints, not only those listed as inflammatory, such as rheumatoid arthritis and acute gout, but also in conditions largely degenerative but with an inflammatory component, such as osteoarthrosis. A large number of non-steroidal anti-inflammatory analgesics are now available (table I; fig. 1).

1. Acetylsalicylic Acid (aspirin)

O-Acetoxybenzoic acid was introduced into medicine in 1899 by Dreser. It is an antipyretic, analgesic substance, with measurable anti-inflammatory properties only apparent in man at full dosage over 4g daily (Boardman and Hart, 1967). It is effective and potentially toxic but may be purchased freely without prescription.

1.1 Actions

Pain relief is effected by a central analgesic action and a peripheral one (Lim, 1966). The types of pain eased are usually those of low intensity, from bone and joint rather than from viscera, but a large variety of pains are eased, ranging from headache and toothache to acute rheumatic fever. Salicylates, according to Vane

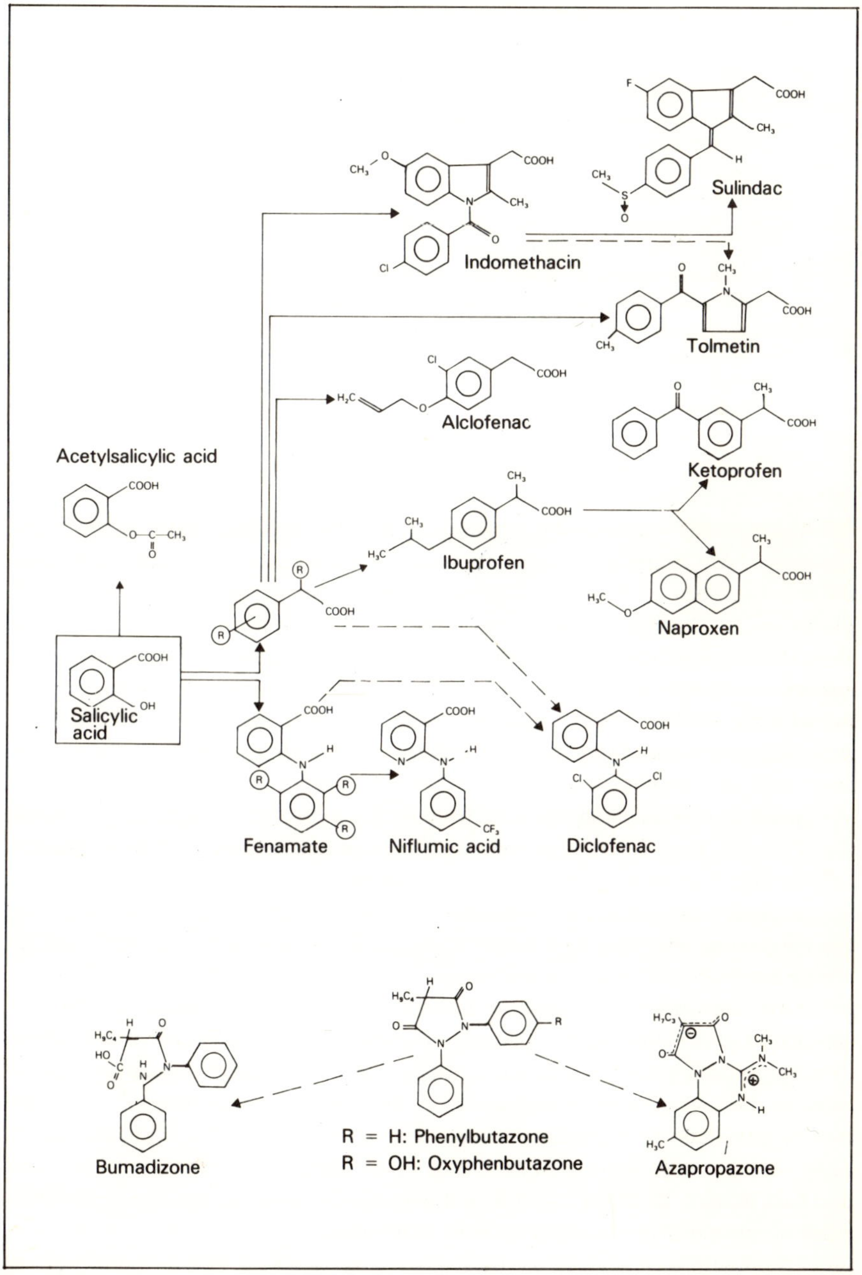

Fig. 1. Structural formulae and inter-relationships of some non-steroidal anti-inflammatory analgesics (after Arznei-Telegramm, p.46 June 1977; by permission).

Table I. Some non-steroidal anti-inflammatory analgesics

1. *Acidic Agents*
    a) Arylcarboxylic acids
        i) Salicylic acids: aspirin, diflunisal
        ii) Anthranilic acids (fenamates): flufenamic, mefenamic, meclofenamic
    b) Aryl alkanoic acids
        i) Aryl acetic acids: alclofenac, diclofenac
        ii) Aryl propionic acids: ibuprofen, flurbiprofen, ketoprofen, naproxen, fenoprofen
        iii) Heteroaryl acetic acids: tolmetin, fenclozic acid
        iv) Indole and indene acetic acids: indomethacin, sulindac
    c) Enolic acids: phenylbutazone, oxyphenbutazone, azapropazone, feprazone

2. *Non-acidic Agents*
    a) Proquazone
    b) Diftalone

(1974), inhibit the synthesis of prostaglandins in inflamed tissues and so prevent sensitisation of pain receptors to substances such as bradykinin, that appear to mediate the pain response. As Morley (1975) points out, however, in assessing the role of mediators in chronic inflammatory responses, different mediators have been emphasised by different scientific disciplines — prostaglandins by pharmacologists, lysosomal enzymes by cell biologists and lymphocytic activation products by immunologists. Morley (1975) regards aspirin as acting not only at the level of prostaglandin production by the macrophage, but possibly on lymphokine action on target cells or lymphokine production by the lymphocyte.

While aspirin can be shown to be truly an anti-inflammatory agent at full dosage (fig. 2), it also has a central analgesic, antipyretic action, possibly at a hypothalamic site; for salicylates at analgesic doses do not cause mental changes or sedation nor sensory changes other than their reduction of pain. The antipyretic action is a non-specific one and fever may be reduced in any condition ranging from a febrile cold to rheumatic fever and miliary tuberculosis.

Salicylates stimulate respiration directly and indirectly, increasing oxygen consumption and carbon dioxide production in animals and man. The increased carbon dioxide production further stimulates respiration, but increased alveolar ventilation balances this and the arterial carbon dioxide tension remains unchanged. Salicylates directly stimulate the respiratory centre, causing hyperventilation with increase in depth and rate of respiration. Therapeutic doses change the electrolyte pattern and acid-base balance, initiating an extra- and intracellular respiratory alkalosis, compensated for promptly by renal excretion of bicarbonate.

Overdosage with salicylates causes initially overbreathing with increased respiration rate and respiratory alkalosis occurs. Plasma salicylate levels of 2.5mmol/L (35mg/100ml) are usually associated in man with hyperventilation and marked hy-

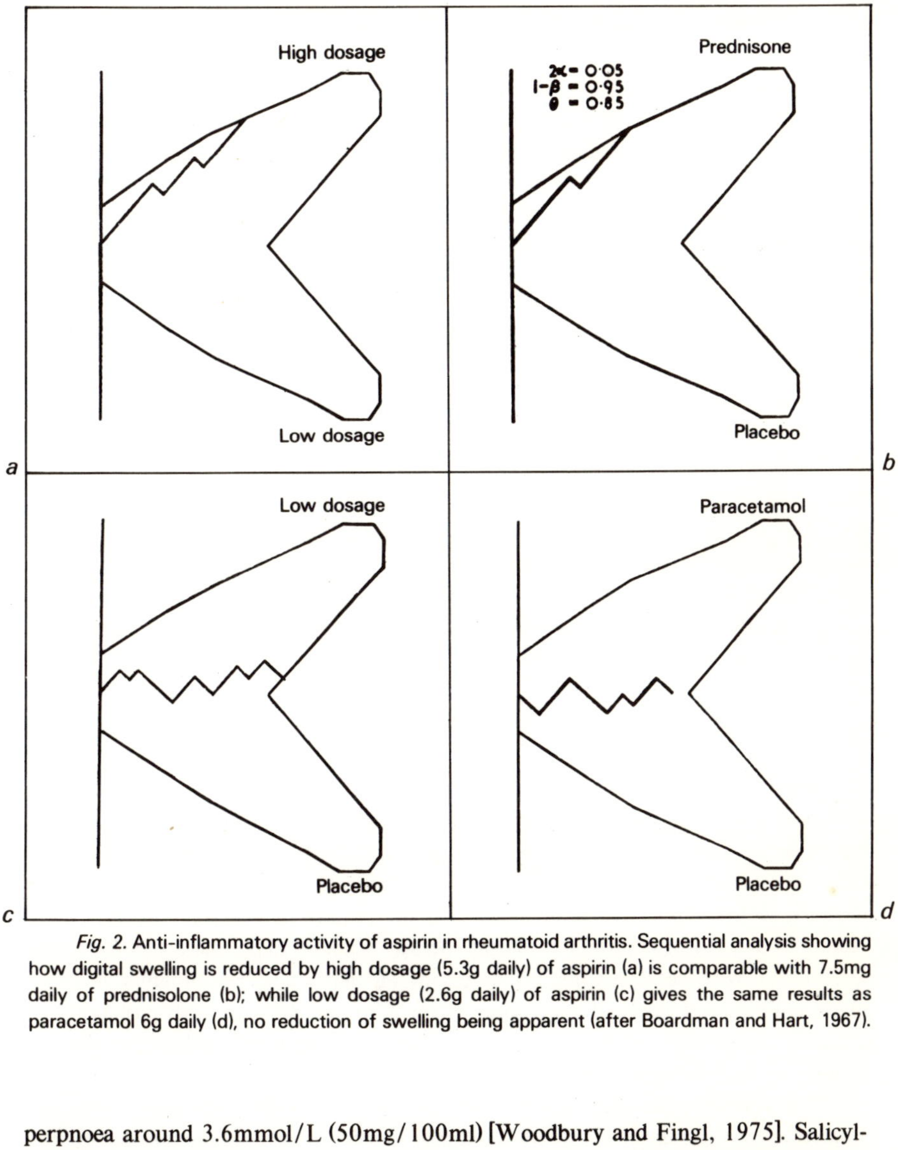

Fig. 2. Anti-inflammatory activity of aspirin in rheumatoid arthritis. Sequential analysis showing how digital swelling is reduced by high dosage (5.3g daily) of aspirin (a) is comparable with 7.5mg daily of prednisolone (b); while low dosage (2.6g daily) of aspirin (c) gives the same results as paracetamol 6g daily (d), no reduction of swelling being apparent (after Boardman and Hart, 1967).

perpnoea around 3.6mmol/L (50mg/100ml) [Woodbury and Fingl, 1975]. Salicylates after prolonged exposure or in excessive dosage have a depressant effect on the medulla and vasomotor depression may result in circulatory collapse and central respiratory paralysis. Continued increase in carbon dioxide production leads to respiratory acidosis and the pulmonary oedema induced by high doses of salicylate limits gaseous exchange in the alveoli and worsens the respiratory acidosis. In infants and children, early overbreathing with respiratory alkalosis may be (and usually is) easily missed. The blood pH and plasma bicarbonate concentration drop but the P_{CO_2} levels remain normal or near normal. The picture is that of a combined respiratory *and* metabolic acidosis (Woodbury and Fingl, 1975; Tenney and Miller, 1955).

Aspirin at doses of 4g a day decreases the plasma iron concentration and shortens the erythrocyte survival time and can cause mild haemolysis in those individuals with a glucose-6-phosphate dehydrogenase deficiency. Aspirin also prolongs the bleeding time, and both *in vitro* and *in vivo,* inhibits many platelet functions: a single dose of aspirin may inhibit platelet aggregation and prolong the bleeding time for several days (Mustard and Packham, 1970; O'Reilly, 1971; Scharrer, 1975).

1.2 Absorption, Distribution and Elimination

Absorption is rapid, partly from the stomach but mostly from the upper small intestine: aspirin is absorbed from the stomach as rapidly as is alcohol and appreciable plasma concentrations are attained within 30 minutes with peak levels after single doses occurring in about 2 hours. A number of factors affect the rate of absorption of aspirin — for instance, the disintegration and dissolution rates of tablets; the physical activity or inactivity of the patient at the time; gastric emptying time; the pH at the mucosal surfaces.

After absorption, aspirin is rapidly distributed throughout all body tissues. It can be detected in the cerebrospinal fluid, the synovial and peritoneal fluid and in saliva and milk and it readily crosses the placenta. It is not secreted in the gastric juice and only very small amounts can be detected in sweat, faeces or bile and it does not accumulate in pathological fluids, such as joint effusions.

Aspirin is mainly absorbed as such but some is hydrolysed in the gastro-intestinal tract and liver, entering the systemic circulation as salicylic acid. Aspirin itself can be detected for only a short time in the plasma after ingestion and concentrations rarely exceed 2mg/100ml (0.14mmol/L) at ordinary therapeutic dose levels. Aspirin is pharmacologically active as such and does not require hydrolysis to salicylic acid. About 50 to 90% of salicylate in routine therapy is bound to plasma proteins, mostly to albumin; with decreased binding occurring at higher dose levels. Thus, in rheumatic conditions associated with low serum albumin, such as active rheumatoid arthritis, a relatively high proportion of free salicylate is present in the plasma. Aspirin as such is bound only to a limited extent.

Salicylates are excreted mainly in the urine, with excretion starting soon after administration, the rate of elimination depending on the dose. Most of a given dose usually can be recovered as free unaltered salicylate, or as metabolites, the result of biotransformation in many tissues, but mostly the liver. The major pathways of metabolism of salicylate are limited at high dosages (explaining why small adjustments of aspirin dosage may be sufficient to eliminate toxic symptoms yet maintain therapeutic plasma salicylate levels). Much depends on the pH of the urine for the rate of clearance of salicylate. Being a weak organic acid, the clearance of salicylate is higher in alkaline than acid urine. Use is made of this in management of severe salicylate poisoning when forced alkaline diuresis is employed to hasten removal of the drug.

The dependence on urine pH for rate of clearance is also important in relation to certain drug interactions with salicylate. Thus, therapeutic doses of antacids such as aluminium and magnesium hydroxides, and sodium bicarbonate markedly decrease plasma levels of salicylate, as a consequence of increased renal clearance caused by the rise in urinary pH, so that therapeutic plasma concentrations may never be maintained.

1.3 Drug Interactions

The scope for interactions of aspirin with other drugs is potentially great (table II), but fortunately, interactions are seldom clinically important. Nevertheless, in the use of a drug which can be taken freely by the patient without prescription, it is important to know of the potential interaction problems. Aspirin in low dosage elevates serum uric acid levels, but at dosage in the order of 5g daily acts as a uricosuric agent. In general, the plasma levels of salicylate are not greatly affected by other drugs except corticosteroids. Concurrent administration of steroids and aspirin decreases plasma salicylate levels due to a more rapid rate of salicylate metabolism, particularly in males, such that therapeutic plasma concentrations of salicylate may not be attained (Graham et al., 1977). Klinenberg and Miller (1965) showed that a decrease in corticosteroid dosage in 4 patients resulted in increased plasma salicylate levels in all cases, with symptoms of salicylate intoxication in one. Concurrent administration of aspirin may lower plasma levels of indomethacin, fenoprofen and naproxen, but usually with no great change in the patients' symptoms.

1.4 Side-effects

Headaches, dizziness and tinnitus are common, particularly at continued high dosage, with difficulty in hearing, dimness of vision, mental confusion, hyperventilation, sweating, thirst and a number of other side-effects. Epigastric distress, nausea, anorexia and vomiting may occur, and are more common at high dosage. Muir (1963) concluded that 1 in 15 patients developed dyspepsia on aspirin and Brooks and Buchanan (1976) found that 30% could not tolerate the drug because of dyspepsia. Haemorrhage and perforation may occur. A pustular acneiform rash may be seen, usually after at least a weeks therapy.

Therapeutic overdosage may more readily occur in children, where severe acid-base and electrolyte disturbances may be missed, as headache and tinnitus are relatively less common; hypoglycaemia is also more common in children. A toxic encephalopathy due to salicylates may be difficult to differentiate from chorea or rheumatoid encephalopathy.

Table II. Potential drug interactions with aspirin

Drug	Possible effect (importance and occurrence depends on circumstances of use)
Alcohol	Increased gastrointestinal irritation with risk of gastric haemorrhage
Aminosalicylic acid (PAS)	Increased risk of salicylism. More likely with large doses
Ammonium chloride Ascorbic acid	Increased plasma salicylate levels due to decreased urinary clearance
Antacids	Decreased plasma salicylate levels due to increased urinary clearance. Therapeutic plasma levels may not be maintained.
Anticoagulants	Increased risk of gastric haemorrhage with both oral anticoagulants and heparin
Antidepressants	Plasma levels and side-effects of nortriptyline and imipramine increased
Antidiabetic drugs (oral)	Increased hypoglycaemic effect with sulphonylureas and large doses of aspirin
Corticosteroids	Accumulation of salicylate with toxicity when long-term steroid therapy withdrawn and dose of aspirin not reduced
Methotrexate	Activity of methotrexate increased
Spironolactone	Possible inhibition of natriuresis
Uricosuric agents	Low doses of aspirin inhibit uricosuric action of probenecid, sulphinpyrazone and phenylbutazone

Although aspirin is regularly associated with blood loss in the alimentary tract, the amounts are usually small and there is usually no correlation with dyspeptic symptoms.

Hypersensitivity reactions are not common, but may occasionally be severe and even fatal, as in acute asthma and anaphylactic reactions, with swelling of skin, periorbital tissues and face, intestine and upper respiratory oedema. Aspirin hypersensitivity may occur after taking only small amounts of the drug, often in a compound tablet, and cannot be foretold by skin testing. True aspirin hypersensitivity is rare, but occurs more commonly than with other salicylate preparations. Many aspirin-sensitive patients also react to indomethacin and ibuprofen.

Aspirin affects platelet function and may occasionally cause purpura or other haemorrhagic manifestations.

1.5 Clinical Use

Of the rheumatic diseases, aspirin is usually considered first choice in rheumatic fever, rheumatoid arthritis (if tolerated), Still's disease (juvenile rheumatoid arthritis), most seronegative arthropathies and most soft tissue lesions, but it is of relatively little help in the treatment of acute gout and severe ankylosing spondylitis. It is of only modest help in the control of most pains caused by osteoarthrosis.

For painful episodes in the day in any rheumatic disorder, aspirin may be used in individual doses of 0.6 to 1g as required, purely as an analgesic. To exert an anti-inflammatory effect, regular dosage every 3 to 4 hours is necessary; total dosage being around 4 to 6g daily. The aim of dosage is to use the lowest effective level, which is often the highest tolerated. Only about half the patients who tolerate lower dosage will continue at the higher dosage of 4 to 6g daily for many weeks, and many of these experience troublesome side-effects. For this reason, propionic acid derivatives such as naproxen and fenoprofen are now often preferred for initial anti-inflammatory therapy in rheumatoid arthritis (see chapt. I; sect. 3).

For optimum anti-inflammatory effect in patients with rheumatoid arthritis, plasma salicylate concentrations of 15 to 30mg/100ml (1.1 to 2.2mmol/L) are required, but there is great individual variation in effect and tolerance. Tinnitus, a reasonably reliable index of plasma levels in those adults with normal hearing, occurs at different plasma levels in different patients, salicylate concentrations ranging from 20 to 46mg/100ml (1.4 to 3.3mmol/L) with total daily doses of 3.6 to 10.8g (Mongan et al., 1973).

1.6 Preparations

Whatever preparation is used, dosage is of the same order as that described above. Preparations available include the following:

1) Aspirin tablet (300mg)
2) Soluble aspirin tablets (calcium aspirin) 300mg, with calcium carbonate, anhydrous citric acid and saccharin sodium
3) Aloxiprin, a polymeric condensation compound of aluminium oxide and aspirin, tablets 600mg; equivalent to 500mg aspirin
4) Sustained release aspirin (microgranular), each microgranule coated with inert methyl cellulose, 500mg tablets. Various other sustained release preparations are available
5) Benorylate, 4-acetamido-2-acetoxy benzoate, is a paracetamol (acetaminophen) ester of aspirin. The drug is absorbed from the gastrointestinal tract as the intact molecule and is then rapidly broken down into its component substances. It is given in suspension, 2 to 4g twice daily, and is also available as tablets containing 750mg; dosage being 1.5g 3 times daily.

Aspirin suppositories are available in some European countries but are not popular elsewhere. Mixtures, powders and suspensions are likely to deteriorate and prove more toxic to the gastrointestinal tract and they are no longer recommended. There are also available a large number of compound tablets and some aspirin preparations which are enteric coated, glycinated, buffered, or coated with paracetamol (acetaminophen). Only buffered aspirin preparations have been convincingly shown to reduce faecal blood loss, but adequate buffering causes rapid renal elimination and therefore these types of formulation are of little use in long-term therapy (Cooke, 1976).

1.7 Use of Aspirin in Childhood

The accepted daily dose of aspirin for the management in childhood of juvenile chronic polyarthritis (Still's disease, juvenile rheumatoid arthritis) is 80mg/kg body weight, given in divided doses (see further chapter XIX). Special preparations for children (e.g. glycinated aspirin) are not particularly helpful, as above the age of 2 or 3 years children can usually tolerate soluble aspirin or aloxiprin dissolved in water, while at an older age they are perfectly able to swallow ordinary enteric coated aspirin. The dosage of benorylate should be 200mg/kg body weight in 2 divided doses per day. It is wise to check that these dosages give an adequate plasma salicylate level (25mg/100ml or 1.8mmol/L).

In the systemic phase of Still's disease, fever is a serious problem and it may then be necessary to give 100mg/kg of aspirin or even more to control this, but when such dose levels are used the child should be watched carefully for evidence of hyperventilation. In any event, it is advisable in a sick child to check the plasma level occasionally as children rarely complain of tinnitus or nausea, although with plasma levels of 44mg/100ml (3.2mmol/L), hyperventilation or vomiting can occur. Symptomatically, gastrointestinal side-effects are extremely rare in children, although occult bleeding does occur. Raised transaminases have been recorded not infrequently when high dosage of aspirin is given, but evidence of permanent liver damage has not been recorded (Athreya et al., 1975).

In rheumatic fever, aspirin in adequate dosage, 100mg/kg body weight given over 24 hours has a dramatic effect on fever and joint symptoms. It has no effect on carditis and, indeed, in the presence of cardiac enlargement or severe mitral valve disease, is contraindicated as fluid retention can occur, causing cardiac embarrassment. Transient rises of transaminase may also be seen in rheumatic fever (see further chapter XVIII).

1.8 Cautions

Aspirin should be used with extreme caution in patients with gastric lesions or on anticoagulants. Pregnancy is not a contraindication as there is no evidence that therapeutic doses cause damage to the fetus, but prolonged high dosage may prolong the length of gestation and labour, probably due to inhibition of prostaglandin synthesis. Small doses of aspirin oppose the uricosuric action of probenecid and sulphinpyrazone.

Contraindications: Known aspirin hypersensitivity. Active peptic ulceration. Cross reactivity may occur with other drugs (e.g. indomethacin).

2. Phenylbutazone

Phenylbutazone is 3,5 dioxo-1,2-diphenyl-4m-butylpyrazolidine, a pyrazolone derivative. It has anti-inflammatory, analgesic and antipyretic properties in animals and man.

2.1 Actions

Phenylbutazone inhibits the biosynthesis of prostaglandins, uncouples oxidative phosphorylation and inhibits ATP-dependent biosynthesis of mucopolysaccharide sulphates in cartilage. It has also a mild uricosuric effect by diminishing tubular reabsorption of uric acid; lower concentrations of the drug have the opposite effect, inhibiting tubular secretion of uric acid and so causing urate retention (Domenjoz, 1960; 1966).

Phenylbutazone causes considerable sodium chloride and water retention and may precipitate heart failure and acute pulmonary oedema in those so predisposed. It causes a fall in urinary output and may induce oedema. Indeed, in the treatment of acute gout, although pain may be relieved dramatically, swelling in the affected area may remain unchanged for this reason (Smyth and Percy, 1973). As a result of this reduction in urine volume, plasma volume may increase, often considerably, hence the dangers of giving the drug to patients with borderline or definite congestive cardiac failure. Potassium excretion is not affected: the retention of sodium and chloride appears to be due to a direct effect of phenylbutazone on the renal tubules. On withdrawing the drug, a compensatory diuresis offloads the excess of sodium and chloride and the expansion of plasma volume returns to normal. These fluid changes are enough in some cases to cause apparent anaemia which disappears after diuresis. Water loading may be controlled, if necessary, by concurrent administration of diuretics.

Phenylbutazone may reduce the uptake of iodine by the thyroid, apparently by a direct effect on that gland, and so may inhibit synthesis of organic iodine compounds. Goitres may, therefore, coccasionally be seen and even frank myxoedema. Phenylbutazone inhibits enzymes of the Krebs cycle and chromosomal damage has been reported by some workers (Stevenson et al., 1971) but others (Walker et al., 1975) found no such changes.

2.2 Absorption, Distribution and Elimination

Phenylbutazone is rapidly and completely absorbed from the gastrointestinal tract and peak plasma concentrations are reached in 2 hours. At usual dose levels, 98% is bound to plasma proteins; higher doses, by increasing plasma levels, may diminish the albumin bound fraction to around 90%. This also means that diseases which alter total drug plasma levels may lead to secondary changes in protein binding. For example, certain liver diseases increase the fraction of free phenylbutazone by 400 to 500%. Phenylbutazone has a low distribution volume of 0.02 to 0.15L/kg. The plasma half-life of phenylbutazone is 29 to 175 hours and is dose-dependent.

The two main metabolites produced by biotransformation in the liver are γ-hydroxyphenylbutazone and oxyphenbutazone which is active and used in therapy (section 3). Hydroxyphenylbutazone has a plasma half-life of about 12 hours and has a marked uricosuric but little antirheumatic or sodium loading effect. Excretion of phenylbutazone and metabolites via the kidneys is slow, as binding to plasma proteins limits glomerular filtration. Only a trace of unchanged phenylbutazone is present in the urine, with 4% of the dose as oxyphenbutazone and about 15% as the uricosuric metabolite II.

2.3 Drug Interactions

Drug interactions are very important. Phenylbutazone has the potential to inhibit the hepatic metabolism and renal excretion of certain drugs, which combined with its ability to displace some highly bound acidic drugs (e.g. warfarin, tolbutamide, chlorpropamide) from plasma albumin binding sites, greatly increases the risk of important drug interactions. Thus, phenylbutazone predictably and markedly enhances the activity of oral coumarin anticoagulants and oral sulphonylurea hypoglycaemic drugs such as tolbutamide and chlorpropamide. Dose requirements of warfarin can be reduced by as much as 50 to 75% with combined phenylbutazone administration and dangerous bleeding episodes have occurred (Koch-Weser and Sellers, 1971). Profound hypoglycaemic coma has been reported following concurrent use of phenylbutazone with acetohexamide, carbutamide, chlorpropamide or tolbutamide, and fatalities have occurred (Hansen and Christensen, 1977). In some patients, phenylbutazone may inhibit the hepatic metabolism of phenytoin and increase plasma levels to the toxic range (Kutt, 1975).

The salt and water retaining effect of phenylbutazone (section 2.1) may lead to inhibition of the action of diuretics and antihypertensive drugs; loss of blood pressure control has been noted. Displacement of plasma protein-bound (globulin) thyroid hormone by phenylbutazone may interfere with the interpretation of thyroid function tests. The anion exchange resin cholestyramine, used in certain hyperlipoproteinaemic disorders, leads to reduced absorption of phenylbutazone taken orally at the same time; if possible, the drugs should be given an hour or more apart.

2.4 Side-effects

There is considerable variation in tolerance of phenylbutazone in different patients: around 20 to 30% of patients note some undesirable effect and the drug will have to be discontinued in about half of these patients. Nausea, vomiting and epigastric discomfort may occur; diarrhoea less commonly. Skin reactions are not uncommon. Peptic ulceration, sometimes with haemorrhage or perforation may occur, as may ulcerative stomatitis (usually without concurrent changes in the blood count), and hypersensitivity reactions like serum sickness and hepatitis. The salt and water retaining effects have been discussed above, as have the dangers of interaction with certain other drugs given concurrently.

All these effects have been freely appreciated since phenylbutazone was introduced in 1952. Blood dyscrasias, however, though less common, are more dangerous. In Great Britain, about 25 patients are reported to the Ministry of Health as dying from the haematological effects of phenylbutazone and oxyphenbutazone each year, but the real figure is probably greater and may be nearer twice this figure. Most of the patients are women over 60 years of age and most are on continuous therapy, usually for osteoarthrosis. Nevertheless, a few deaths have been reported in younger patients on shorter courses of treatment. These deaths are due usually to hypoplastic anaemia with suppression of all cell series, including platelets, and the resulting haemorrhage may prove fatal. Suppression of individual cell series manifesting as agranulocytosis, neutropenia and thrombocytopenia is occasionally seen, and these carry a lower mortality than complete aplasia, but around half of all cases reported with blood dyscrasias prove fatal. Acute sensitivity reactions and fatal blood changes from short courses of therapy are very rare. Fowler (1967) and Fowler and Faragher (1977) point out that 87% of patients who develop agranulocytosis do so within 3 months of starting treatment as compared with only 30% of patients with aplastic anaemia. Around 50% of patients with aplastic anaemia develop this complication after at least 1 years treatment.

Although it is wise to do full blood counts and platelet counts before initial long-term therapy and periodically thereafter, these blood changes may occur suddenly between routine counts, even if performed every 3 to 4 weeks, so they carry no absolute assurance of avoidance of this complication. Although such fatal reactions occur rarely, Inman (1977) estimates a death rate of 16.7 per 100,000 patient years of treatment for phenylbutazone and 40 per 100,000 patient years of treatment for oxyphenbutazone; these drugs probably cause more than one third of all drug-induced blood dyscrasias in Great Britain excluding cancer chemotherapy (Inman, 1977).

The pyrazolones continue to be widely used because they are effective anti-inflammatory, analgesic and antipyretic agents with an even action over the 24 hours which is of benefit in diseases such as rheumatoid arthritis where pain tends to be recurring or chronic and inflammatory features present throughout most hours of the day and night; they are cheap; they are usually well tolerated; and many patients prefer them. Born, as it were, out of amidopyrine, in combination with which under the name Irgapyrine, phenylbutazone first appeared in the United Kingdom, it shares with that drug a tendency to cause blood dyscrasias, though of a different nature from the parent substance.

2.5 Clinical Use

Phenylbutazone is effective in almost all the rheumatic disorders, particularly in acute gout, ankylosing spondylitis, osteoarthrosis, rheumatoid arthritis and in Reiter's disease and other seronegative arthropathies (Hart, 1953). It has also proved its efficacy in the past in rheumatic fever. Phenylbutazone may also help to control symptoms from prolapsed intervertebral disc, Paget's disease of bone and metastatic malignant disease of bone. Nevertheless, though highly effective, it is wise, because of its side-effects and drug interactions, to use it only where a less potentially dangerous agent fails to control symptoms. It is also wise not to continue its use indefinitely, particularly in patients over the age of 60, without close clinical (patients should be asked to report any unusual symptoms such as rash, fever, sore throat) and haematological control, appreciating the fact that even then blood dyscrasias may occur rapidly and prove fatal. It is also wise not to use phenylbutazone to treat mild conditions such as trivial sports or other injuries where less toxic agents would suffice.

2.6 Dosage

Phenylbutazone is prescribed as 100 and 200mg tablets orally after food. In acute gout, 600 to 800mg is given initially on the first day, reducing dosage as symptoms come under control by 100 to 200mg daily to a maintenance of 200 to 400mg; withdrawing the drug as soon as the attack is over. In chronic arthritic conditions, 100 to 400mg daily is usual; with every effort to keep dosage to the lowest effective level. Phenylbutazone should always be given with or after food. Enteric coated and antacid incorporated tablets are available, as are suppositories of 250mg. It is effective, though sometimes painful, given by intramuscular injection of 200mg of the sodium salt with lignocaine hydrochloride.

2.7 Cautions

Initial and periodic blood counts are advisable, including platelet counts (see also section 2.4). In chronic dyspepsia, it is wise to avoid phenylbutazone. Similarly, it is best to avoid use of phenylbutazone in patients with renal or hepatic disease, including recent hepatitis.

Contraindications: Cardiac decompensation; peptic ulceration. Phenylbutazone should be avoided in patients receiving oral coumarin anticoagulants or sulphonylurea hypoglycaemic drugs (see section 2.3).

3. Oxyphenbutazone

Oxyphenbutazone, 4-butyl-1-p-hydroxyphenyl-3,5-dioxo-2-phenylpyrazolidine monohydrate is a hydroxy analogue of phenylbutazone and one of its major metabolites. It has the same general properties and the same actions, therapeutic uses, interactions and toxic effects as the parent drug. Although initially it was thought that side-effects might prove less common than with phenylbutazone this has not proved to be so. Pharmacologically, therapeutically and toxicologically it may be regarded as the same substance. It is available as 100mg tablets and 250mg suppositories and as enteric coated 100mg tablets.

4. Indomethacin

Indomethacin is 1-(p-chlorobenzoyl)-5 methoxy-2-methylindole-3-acetic acid. It has anti-inflammatory and antipyretic properties in animals and man, and relieves pain effectively in man in a large range of conditions.

4.1 Actions

Indomethacin inhibits the biosynthesis of prostaglandins, inhibits motility of polymorphonuclear leucocytes and uncouples oxidative phosphorylation in cartilaginous and hepatic mitrochondria. Its therapeutic action begins about 2 hours or less after an oral dose of 25 to 50mg and lasts some 6 hours or more. Indomethacin is, perhaps with phenylbutazone, the most potent non-steroidal anti-inflammatory agent available today and will if tolerated reduce inflammatory swelling and lessen pain in gout and the inflammatory arthropathies (fig. 3) effectively in many cases (Hart and Boardman, 1963, 1965), though it is less effective than the corticosteroids in reducing tissue swelling (Hart and Boardman, 1964).

4.2 Absorption, Distribution and Elimination

After oral ingestion, indomethacin is rapidly and almost completely absorbed from the gastrointestinal tract; peak plasma concentrations occurring within 3 hours in a fasting subject but later after food. It is 92 to 99% bound to plasma proteins and widely distributed in tissues, although concentrations are low in the cerebrospinal fluid. It has a relatively large distribution volume of 0.34 to 1.57L/kg and a plasma half-life of 4 to 12 hours. After absorption, indomethacin is largely converted to inactive metabolites. Some of these metabolites are detected in plasma; free and conjugated metabolites are eliminated in the urine, bile and faeces. 10 to 20% of the drug is excreted unchanged in the urine, in part by tubular secretion, possibly necessitating reduction of dosing in patients with renal failure.

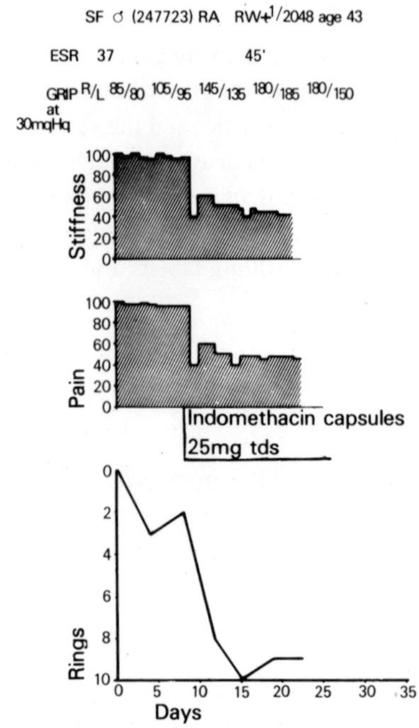

Fig. 3. Anti-inflammatory activity of indomethacin in rheumatoid arthritis. Effect on grip strength, stiffness and pain assessed by the patient, and reduction in digital swelling as measured by jewellers rings (after Hart and Boardman, 1963).

4.3 Drug Interactions

The precise mechanism and clinical significance of reported indomethacin-aspirin interaction is unclear. Recent studies have shown no significant reduction in indomethacin plasma levels following combined administration of aspirin and oral or rectal indomethacin (Brooks et al., 1975; Lindquist et al., 1974). On the other hand, buffered aspirin given at the same time as oral indomethacin, appears to increase the rate of absorption and severity of side-effects of indomethacin (Garnham et al., 1975). Clinical studies also suggest an increased incidence of indomethacin side-effects with combined aspirin-indomethacin therapy (Brooks et al., 1975). In practice, the effect of aspirin on indomethacin is very variable between different patients and its significance difficult to determine.

Concurrent administration of probenecid does, however, increase total plasma concentrations of indomethacin (i.e. unchanged drug + inactive metabolites) and appears to enhance pain relief without increasing indomethacin side-effects (Brooks et al., 1974), but whether reduced dosage of indomethacin is needed is not clear. Indomethacin does not affect the uricosuric action of probenecid, nor does it have any effect on the hypoprothrombinaemic action or plasma levels of warfarin in normal volunteers (Vessel et al., 1975).

4.4 Side-effects

Headaches, vertigo, mental 'muzziness', confusion and a number of other cerebral sensations are dose related and diminish or disappear with reduction of dosage. Gastrointestinal symptoms, abdominal pain, vague discomfort, anorexia or peptic ulceration, sometimes with bleeding and perforation, are not dose related and may occur at any time on any dose. Diffuse gastritis with bleeding may occur, but is rare, as are prepyloric gastric ulcers, which though resembling carcinomatous lesions disappear within 4 to 5 weeks of stopping indomethacin administration.

Blood changes have been reported but are rare, though thrombocytopenia, sometimes with purpura may rarely occur. Severe depression, hallucinations and even psychoses have been reported. Skin rashes are uncommon, as are hypersensitivity reactions such as urticaria, pruritus and asthma. Patients allergic to aspirin may cross-react also with indomethacin. The dangers to children of activating latent septic lesions have been, in the author's opinion, overemphasised. Suppositories of indomethacin may cause anal irritation in some patients, but are well tolerated over long periods by most. The use of suppositories may diminish, but does not entirely prevent, gastrointestinal irritation.

Although a large number of uncommon reactions have been reported, in practice toxic side-effects are mostly cerebral sensations (dose related) and gastrointestinal reactions (not dose related). Patients with impaired renal function are more likely to react adversely to the drug, since elimination is probably prolonged (see section 3.2).

4.5 Clinical Use

Indomethacin is useful throughout almost the entire field of rheumatic disorders, but is most helpful in ankylosing spondylitis, gout, rheumatoid arthritis and osteoarthrosis, particularly of the hip. About 20 to 30 % of patients cannot tolerate it at effective dose levels, but about the same proportion do rather better with it than with most non-steroidal anti-inflammatory analgesics. It is effective in seronegative arthropathies, such as Reiter's disease and psoriatic arthropathy, but it may aggravate ulcerative lesions of stomach or intestine and should in general never be given to patients with peptic ulcers, Crohn's disease or ulcerative colitis. Indomethacin has proved helpful as an anti-inflammatory and pain-relieving drug after orthopaedic operations.

A loading dose given at night is helpful in those disorders such as ankylosing spondylitis and rheumatoid arthritis, where pain is often at its worst at night so preventing normal sleep, and where morning stiffness is a major symptom. In such cases, the indomethacin suppository is particularly useful.

4.6 Dosage

The usual dosage is 25mg 2 to 4 times a day taken orally after or with meals. It is wise to start with a test dose after the evening meal in case the patient proves to be an 'over-reactor'. Taken at night on retiring, 50 to 100mg by mouth with food or as a suppository, indomethacin is often very helpful in relieving nocturnal symptoms. In acute gout, larger doses are necessary, 100mg for night cover and 100 to 150mg in the day in divided dosage after food; dosage being reduced as symptoms abate. Some patients may need even larger doses initially. It is available as capsules of 25 and 50mg and suppositories of 100mg and in some countries as an elixir of 25mg per 5ml.

4.7 Cautions

Headaches and various cerebral sensations may occur early in therapy. There is considerable variation in individual tolerance. Psychiatric disease, Parkinsonism and epilepsy may be exacerbated. Many patients hypersensitive to aspirin cross-react to indomethacin.

Contraindications: Active peptic ulceration. A history of recurrent gastrointestinal erosions.

5. Ibuprofen

Ibuprofen is 2-(4-isobutylphenyl) propionic acid. It was the first of the propionic acid derivatives to be introduced in most countries, and has proved to be very popular. It is an analgesic with minor anti-inflammatory properties. It is so classified because although it has potent anti-inflammatory effects in animal models, in man its anti-inflammatory effect is not striking. Ibuprofen is less effective than the major anti-inflammatory drugs such as high dose aspirin in conditions like rheumatoid arthritis. On the other hand, its analgesic effect is roughly equivalent to that of aspirin and it is therefore effective in non-inflammatory painful rheumatic conditions.

5.1 Absorption, Distribution and Elimination

Ibuprofen is well absorbed from the stomach and has a short plasma half-life of about 2 hours. Absorption is a little slower when the drug is given after food. It is about 99% protein bound and has a low distribution volume of 0.14L/kg. Excretion is via urine and in bile, 10% as unchanged drug and the remainder as inactive metabolites.

5.2 Drug Interactions

Ibuprofen does not appear to affect hepatic drug metabolism and can be given to patients receiving oral coumarin anticoagulants, but it is wise to check the prothrombin time daily for the first several days of combined administration.

5.3 Side-effects

The great advantage of ibuprofen is that it is very well tolerated and it is seldom necessary to withdraw treatment because of troublesome side-effects. It causes strikingly fewer toxic effects than high dose aspirin therapy and more patients are able to continue treatment. It is as well tolerated as naproxen and better tolerated than ketoprofen or fenoprofen. The most common side-effects are epigastric discomfort, nausea and indigestion. Occasional gastrointestinal haemorrhages have been reported. Rashes occur occasionally and exacerbation of asthma has been reported in patients whose asthma was made worse by aspirin. Toxic amblyopia has also been reported, but was rapidly reversible when the drug was withdrawn. Nevertheless, it is wise to stop ibuprofen in any patient who complains of deterioration of vision. Though related to ibufenac, it does not cause jaundice.

5.4 Clinical Use

Ibuprofen is useful in a wide range of rheumatic disorders from the milder cases of rheumatoid arthritis to osteoarthrosis and back pain. It is less suitable for very active rheumatoid arthritis, acute Reiter's disease, acute gout, ankylosing spondylitis and other conditions in which inflammation is prominent.

As with other non-steroidal anti-inflammatory analgesics, there is a striking individual variation in response. Many patients do not respond at all to ibuprofen and some respond very well. It works quickly so that if it has not proved helpful by the end of a week, it is unlikely to do so later.

5.5 Preparations and Dosage

Ibuprofen is available as 200 or 400mg tablets. There is some argument about the correct dosage. Most reported studies of ibuprofen have used 1200mg daily. Doses smaller than this are unlikely to be effective. Evidence that larger doses are more effective is not particularly convincing. It seems that occasional patients may respond better to larger doses and therefore it is best to start with 1,200mg daily and

POM → P.

increase if necessary, reviewing the patient's progress at different dose levels. Ibuprofen can be used in children in doses up to 40mg/kg per day.

5.6 Cautions

Ibuprofen may with caution be given to patients with peptic ulcer and is usually well tolerated. Oral anticoagulants are discussed above. It should be given with caution to patients who have shown hypersensitivity to aspirin or other non-steroidal anti-inflammatory analgesics.

6. Naproxen

Naproxen is (+)-2-(6-methoxy-2-napthyl)-propionic acid. It is one of the more effective propionic acid derivatives. Although it is most appropriately classified in this group, and like other members of the group it has a low incidence of side-effects, it is about as effective as aspirin. It also has the advantage of twice daily administration and may be considered the first choice of the propionic acid derivatives, because it combines greatest effectiveness and lowest incidence of side-effects compared with other members of the group.

6.1 Absorption, Distribution and Elimination

Naproxen is well absorbed from the stomach. The rate of absorption is enhanced by concomitant administration of sodium bicarbonate and reduced by aluminium hydroxide and other antacids; the clinical significance of this remains unknown. Steady state plasma levels of the drug are reached after about 3 days of regular administration. Naproxen is protein bound to the extent of 98 to 99% and has a low distribution volume of 0.09L/kg. Protein binding seems to be saturated at higher plasma concentrations (i.e. at doses above 500mg daily), thereby increasing the fraction of unbound drug available for distribution and elimination, and resulting in accelerated clearance and lower than expected plasma levels. There is little increase in plasma concentrations of naproxen with doses above 500mg daily.

Compared with other propionic acid derivatives, naproxen has a relatively long plasma half-life of 10 to 17 hours, which allows its administration on a twice daily basis. There is no obvious correlation between plasma levels and effectiveness. Naproxen is excreted almost entirely in the urine; either unchanged or largely as the glucuronide conjugate and demethylated naproxen.

6.2 Drug Interactions

Although naproxen is highly protein bound and has a low distribution volume, it can be given to patients taking oral coumarin anticoagulants. Occasional patients may nevertheless show prolongation of prothrombin time, which should be checked daily for the first several days of administration of any such combined therapy. Administration of aspirin leads to a slight reduction of naproxen plasma levels but this is probably insignificant. In most cases it is pointless to give two anti-inflammatory drugs together.

6.3 Side-effects

Naproxen is remarkably free of side-effects. Compared with high doses of aspirin, there is a large reduction in the incidence of side-effects and an increase in the number of patients able to continue treatment. Compared with other propionic acid derivatives, naproxen along with ibuprofen, is among the less toxic. Occasional instances of gastrointestinal bleeding have been reported (Hart and Matts, 1974), and appear to be slightly more common with naproxen than with other propionic acid derivatives, particularly in patients who have had similar side-effects with other non-steroidal anti-inflammatory agents.

The most common side-effects are epigastric discomfort, nausea and indigestion, which occur in about 5 % of patients. They are usually mild and seldom lead to withdrawal of treatment. Rare side-effects include rash, headache and 'light-headedness'.

6.4 Clinical Use

Naproxen is useful for the non-specific or symptomatic treatment of a wide range of rheumatic disorders from rheumatoid arthritis to soft tissue rheumatism and backache. It is perhaps less useful than aspirin in the most active cases of rheumatoid arthritis and less useful than indomethacin and phenylbutazone in ankylosing spondylitis. Although it has been shown to be effective in acute gout, there is no reason why it should replace indomethacin and phenylbutazone in the treatment of this condition. — Eff-

It is important to note that naproxen is effective only in about 60 % of patients with rheumatoid arthritis and that differences between patient responses are much greater than differences between drugs. Naproxen is therefore a most useful drug for a particular subgroup of patients. It takes effect within 24 hours of the start of treatment and a week of therapy is certainly long enough to assess its effectiveness. If it has not worked at this time, it is pointless to continue treatment.

6.5 Preparations and Dosage

Naproxen is available as a 250mg tablet and the usual dosage is 250mg twice daily. A larger dose (500mg) may be useful at night for the relief of morning stiffness.

6.6. Cautions

Naproxen has been given to patients with peptic ulcer and has been well tolerated in most cases (Roth and Boost, 1975). Gastric haemorrhage, however, has been reported in such cases. Anticoagulant therapy is discussed above. Hypersensitivity reactions may occur in patients who have had reactions with other non-steroidal anti-inflammatory analgesics.

7. Fenoprofen

Fenoprofen is the calcium salt of dl-2-(3-phenoxyphenyl) propionic acid. It is one of the more effective propionic acid derivatives. Like other members of the group it has a low incidence of side-effects, and like naproxen is as effective as aspirin.

7.1 Absorption, Distribution and Elimination

Fenoprofen is well absorbed after oral administration. Blood levels of the drug are slightly lower when it is taken with food, but this probably has no clinical significance. Concurrent administration of aspirin also lowers the blood levels slightly. There is no correlation between blood levels and clinical response to fenoprofen. The plasma half-life is short; around 2 hours. More than 99% of the drug is bound to plasma proteins and it has a low distribution volume of 0.08 to 0.11L/kg. The ingested drug is extensively metabolised and the metabolites are rapidly excreted in the urine, mostly in the form of fenoprofen and hydroxyfenoprofen glucuronides.

7.2 Drug Interactions

Fenoprofen can be given to patients taking oral coumarin anticoagulants, although occasional patients may show prolongation of prothrombin time, which should be checked daily for the first several days of administration of both drugs.

7.3 Side-effects

Compared with high dose aspirin, fenoprofen is very well tolerated with fewer side-effects, and many more patients are able to continue treatment. Side-effects which occur are usually mild and seldom lead to withdrawal of treatment. Compared with other propionic acid derivatives, fenoprofen is more likely to cause minor side-effects, especially those of a gastrointestinal nature. Epigastric discomfort, nausea or indigestion occur in about 20% of patients. Epigastric discomfort often follows immediately after taking the capsules and seems to be a little less common with the tablets which are available in the United Kingdom. Antacids may be given to relieve these symptoms. Rare side-effects include rashes and hypersensitivity reactions. Few serious or dangerous side-effects have been reported, but gastrointestinal haemorrhage may occur.

7.4 Clinical Use

Fenoprofen is useful in a wide variety of rheumatic disorders for non-specific or symptomatic therapy. In rheumatoid arthritis it is as effective as full doses of aspirin and it has also been shown to be effective in osteoarthrosis and acute gout. It is most suitable for the less inflammatory conditions like osteoarthrosis and all but the most active cases of rheumatoid arthritis.

Like naproxen, fenoprofen is effective in about 60 % of patients with rheumatoid arthritis. These two drugs are more effective than both ibuprofen and ketoprofen. Fenoprofen takes effect quickly, so that if it has not proved effective after a week, it is unlikely to prove helpful and should be stopped. Differences between patient responses are greater than differences between drugs of the type and fenoprofen is useful in a particular subgroup of patients.

7.5 Preparations and Dosage

Fenoprofen is available as a 300mg capsule or tablet. The usual initial dosage is 2.4g daily in 4 divided doses but in patients who respond well, this can often be reduced to 1.2 or 1.8g daily. For maintenance therapy, the lowest effective dose should be used.

7.6 Cautions

Fenoprofen may possibly be given with caution to some patients with peptic ulcer, though formal studies have not been reported. In general, it is wiser in cases of peptic ulceration to avoid using any non-steroidal anti-inflammatory agent unless it proves essential and absolutely necessary. Anticoagulant therapy is discussed above. Hypersensitivity reactions may occur in patients who have had reactions with other non-steroidal anti-inflammatory analgesics.

8. Ketoprofen

Ketoprofen is 2-(3-benzoylphenyl) propionic acid. It is one of the group of analgesics with minor anti-inflammatory properties, similar in effectiveness to ibuprofen.

8.1 Absorption, Distribution and Elimination

Ketoprofen is well absorbed following oral administration. It has a short plasma half-life of about 2 hours but a much longer synovial fluid half-life, which may be a more useful guide to the time course of the action of the drug. It is rapidly excreted in the urine, mainly in the form of glucuronides.

8.2 Drug Interactions

Ketoprofen can be given to patients receiving oral coumarin anticoagulants but it is wise to check the prothrombin time daily for the first several days of combined administration of the drugs. No other interactions are known.

8.3 Side-effects

Ketoprofen is better tolerated than high dose aspirin but not as well tolerated as naproxen and ibuprofen. The most common side-effects are those arising from the upper gastrointestinal tract, with epigastric discomfort, nausea and flatulence the most frequent complaints. Occasional side-effects include rashes and hypersensitivity reactions.

8.4 Clinical Use

Ketoprofen is useful in a wide range of rheumatic disorders, particularly those in which inflammation is less prominent. It is therefore likely to be particularly useful in the less active cases of rheumatoid arthritis, osteoarthrosis or soft tissue rheumatism. Although it may appear that, among propionic acid derivatives, ketoprofen has no obvious advantages, individual variation in responsiveness does make this a useful compound for a small subgroup of patients. There are patients who prefer naproxen, patients who prefer fenoprofen or ibuprofen, and patients who prefer ketoprofen. It takes effect quickly and need only be given for a week to determine whether a patient is likely to respond.

8.5 Preparations and Dosage

Ketoprofen is available as 50mg capsules and the usual dosage is 50mg 3 times daily. In some countries, it is also available for injection and as a 100mg suppository. The suppository dosage form may be useful at night for relief of morning stiffness and in patients who cannot tolerate oral dosage.

8.6 Cautions

There is no reported work on the use of ketoprofen in patients with peptic ulcer and this should therefore be undertaken with caution (see section 6.6). Patients who have developed hypersensitivity reactions to aspirin or other non-steroidal anti-inflammatory analgesics may react similarly to ketoprofen.

9. Alclofenac

Alclofenac is 4-allyloxy-3-chlorophenylacetic acid. It is one of a group of analgesics with minor anti-inflammatory properties and as such resembles ibuprofen and other propionic acid derivatives. It has been claimed to have a long-term advantage of reducing the activity of the disease itself in addition to analgesic and anti-inflammatory properties, but this awaits confirmation. Rashes, which are sometimes serious, are a disadvantage.

9.1 Absorption, Distribution and Elimination

Alclofenac appears to be variably absorbed following oral administration. Plasma levels are decreased if the drug is taken with or shortly after a meal. Drug concentrations in synovial fluid are higher than in plasma sampled at the same time. About 90 to 99% of the drug is bound to plasma proteins and the distribution volume is low; 0.07 to 0.1L/kg. The plasma half-life is about 2.5 hours, ranging between 1.5 and 5.5. hours. Most of the ingested dose is excreted in the urine as alclofenac glucuronide with smaller amounts of unchanged alclofenac and hydroxylated glucuronides. In some patients, a significant proportion (up to 50%) of the administered dose is excreted unchanged in the urine. Dosage may therefore need to be modified in patients with renal failure. Significant amounts of the drug are excreted in the faeces in some patients.

9.2 Drug Interactions

Alclofenac may theoretically enhance the activity of oral coumarin anticoagulants and oral sulphonylurea hypoglycaemic drugs.

9.3 Side-effects

The most important adverse reaction is skin rash. Gastrointestinal problems are unusual with this drug and apart from these and occasional hypersensitivity reactions, no other important side-effects have been reported.

Skin reactions occur in about 10% of patients given alclofenac tablets and 2% of those given capsules (Hort, 1975). They occur within the first 10 days of treatment and are usually 'allergic' in type. They seem to be particularly common in patients with a history of penicillin allergy. About 10% of rashes are severe and associated with some systemic upset. Hypersensitivity angiitis with purpuric and petechial rashes (Billings et al., 1974), epistaxis, haemoptysis and haematuria have been reported. Patients should be warned to stop the drug immediately if a rash develops.

9.4 Clinical Use

Alclofenac is effective as symptomatic treatment in a wide range of rheumatic disorders. It is an alternative to propionic acid derivatives for patients in whom inflammation is not prominent.

An additional action for alclofenac has been claimed in rheumatoid arthritis. Studies from one group (Aylward et al., 1975) have shown a 'penicillamine-like' effect with gradual amelioration of manifestations of rheumatoid arthritis over a 6 month period, reduction in ESR, rheumatoid factor and immunoglobulins and less radiological deterioration than in patients receiving indomethacin. These findings await confirmation.

9.5 Preparations and Dosage

Alclofenac is available as a 500mg capsule. The usual initial dose is 1g 3 times daily but a maintenance dose of 500mg 3 times daily may be sufficient.

9.6 Cautions

Alclofenac should be used with caution in patients with peptic ulcer since formal studies have not been carried out. Similarly, it should be used with caution in patients receiving oral anticoagulants or oral sulphonylurea hypoglycaemic drugs.

10. Tolmetin

Tolmetin is 1-methyl-5-p-toluoylpyrrole-2 acetic acid. It has some chemical similarities to indomethacin but behaves in man more like propionic acid derivatives and is therefore classified as an analgesic with minor anti-inflammatory properties. Like other drugs of this class, it has a big advantage over aspirin in the incidence of gastric side-effects and in the number of patients able to continue treatment.

10.1 Absorption, Distribution and Elimination

Tolmetin is well absorbed following oral administration and has a relatively short plasma half-life of about 1 hour. It is 99% bound to plasma proteins and has a low distribution volume of 0.10L/kg. It is excreted in the urine; mainly as tolmetin glucuronide or as an inactive dicarboxylic acid metabolite and its glucuronide, with small amounts as unchanged drug.

10.2 Drug Interactions

Tolmetin can be given with oral coumarin anticoagulants but it is wise to check the prothrombin time daily for the first several days of combined administration of the drugs. Concurrent administration of aspirin reduces plasma concentrations of tolmetin, but the clinical significance is uncertain.

10.3 Side-effects

Side-effects of tolmetin are mainly of a gastrointestinal nature and occur in about 30% of patients treated. Studies comparing tolmetin and aspirin have shown an important advantage for tolmetin; aspirin caused 50% more side-effects in one study (Ehrlich and Roth, 1976). Withdrawal from treatment with tolmetin is unusual but may be necessary in about 10% of all patients because of gastric problems; nausea, epigastric pain and indigestion are the most frequent complaints. Less common side-effects include headaches or dizziness, which occur in about 15% of patients but are usually mild and not troublesome. Rashes, oedema and hypersensitivity reactions occur occasionally.

10.4 Clinical Use

Tolmetin is useful in a wide range of rheumatic disorders as a well-tolerated drug for relief of symptoms. It is probably especially useful in diseases in which inflammation is not prominent. Its effects in rheumatoid arthritis are comparable with those of full doses of aspirin.

10.5 Preparation and Dosage

Tolmetin is available as a 200mg tablet. Doses of about 1200mg in 4 divided doses daily are required in rheumatoid arthritis, though individual patients may require as little as 800mg daily or as much as 1600mg daily.

10.6 Cautions

Studies to date suggest that tolmetin is not well tolerated by peptic ulcer patients and should be used with caution. Oral anticoagulants are discussed above.

11. Sulindac

Sulindac is an indene derivative of indomethacin which appears to have effects similar to indomethacin in the treatment of rheumatoid and osteoarthrosis, but without some of the characteristic side-effects. It is given on a twice daily basis.

11.1 Absorption, Distribution and Elimination

Sulindac itself is a sulphoxide. It is well absorbed following oral administration and has a plasma half-life of about 7 hours. Absorption is slightly delayed when the drug is taken with food but this is unlikely to be significant clinically. Once absorbed, the sulphoxide is enterohepatically recycled and converted in the lumen of the gut (Duggan et al., 1977) to two other compounds, the sulphone and sulphide. The sulphide, which is also recycled, appears to be important because it is pharmacologically active and in animal models of inflammation it appears to account for a major part of the action of the administered drug. The sulphide has an even longer plasma half-life of 18 hours and because of this, sulindac can be given on a twice daily basis. The sulphone is not active as an anti-inflammatory agent. Sulindac and its sulphone metabolite are excreted in the urine and bile, either unchanged or mainly as the glucuronide conjugates. The active sulphide metabolite is excreted in the faeces and not in the urine.

11.2 Drug Interactions

Sulindac can be given to patients receiving oral coumarin anticoagulants but it is wise to check the prothrombin time daily for the first several days of combined administration of the drugs. It slightly reduces the uricosuric effect of probenecid but this is unlikely to be important.

11.3 Side-effects

Sulindac causes less side-effects than aspirin. Those side-effects which occur tend to be mild and seldom lead to withdrawal of treatment. It does not cause headaches (as indomethacin does) and is much less likely than aspirin to cause gastric side-effects. Constipation, epigastric pain and nausea are nevertheless the most common problems, occurring in about 25 % of patients. Greater experience will probably be required to document the less common side-effects.

11.4 Clinical Use

Sulindac is as effective as aspirin in rheumatoid arthritis and osteoarthrosis. It is more effective than ibuprofen and comparable with naproxen. Surprisingly, it appears to be significantly less effective than indomethacin and phenylbutazone in ankylosing spondylitis. It is therefore a useful alternative to indomethacin in conditions other than ankylosing spondylitis. It has also been shown to be effective in acute gout and soft tissue rheumatism.

11.5 Preparations and Dosage

Sulindac is available as a 100mg tablet. A dose of 200mg twice daily is usually required in severe rheumatoid arthritis and represents a satisfactory starting dose for other conditions. The dose can often be reduced to 200mg daily in osteoarthrosis and milder conditions and it should be given in the lowest effective maintenance dose.

11.6 Cautions

The drug should only be given with extreme caution to patients with peptic ulcer until further experience is obtained. Anticoagulant therapy has been mentioned above.

12. Flufenamic Acid

Flufenamic acid (n-γγγ-trifluoro-m-tolyl anthranilic acid), is an analgesic, anti-inflammatory agent with antipyretic properties in the experimental animal. However, Brooks and Buchanan (1976) consider an anti-inflammatory effect in man with flufenamic acid and another anthranilate, mefenamic acid, as still unproven; mefenamic acid in particular seems to have only slight anti-inflammatory activity in arthritic disorders in man.

12.1 Absorption, Distribution and Elimination

After oral administration, peak plasma levels of flufenamic acid occur about 3 to 6 hours following ingestion. A secondary peak in blood levels after about 8 hours is due to the presence of hydroxylated metabolites, probably as a result of enterohepatic circulation. Plasma protein binding is almost complete. Excretion is via the urine (around 55%) as unchanged drug, glucuronide conjugate and hydroxylated glucuronides, as well as via the faeces (around 36%).

12.2 Side-effects

Side-effects are nausea, vomiting, diarrhoea (10% of cases or more) and epigastric discomfort. Sensitivity type rashes are unusual. Haemolytic anaemia has been reported with mefenamic acid (Holmes, 1967).

12.3 Clinical Use

Flufenamic acid may be considered in osteoarthrosis and rheumatoid arthritis where propionic acid derivatives prove ineffective or are poorly tolerated.

12.4 Preparations and Dosage

Flufenamic acid is available as 100 and 200mg capsules. Dosage ranges from 300 to 600mg daily in 3 divided doses, preferably with food. Mefenamic acid is available in 250mg capsules, daily dosage being 1.5g.

12.5 Cautions

Flufenamic acid may theoretically enhance the activity of oral coumarin anticoagulants and oral sulphonylurea hypoglycaemic drugs. Gastrointestinal upsets necessitate reduction of dosage or discontinuance of the drug. Enzyme levels of SGOT and SGPT may rise on therapy. Both flufenamic and mefenamic acid cause bronchoconstriction in aspirin-sensitive asthmatics. Flufenamic acid should not be used in patients with peptic ulcer or other ulcerative lesions of the gastrointestinal tract (e.g. ulcerative colitis).

13. Azapropazone

Azapropazone is 5-(dimethylamino)-9-methyl-2-propyl)-(1H-pyrazolo(1-2-α) (1,2,4)benzotriazine-1,3(2H)dione dihydrate. Although its chemical structure resembles that of phenylbutazone (fig. 1), its actions and side-effects more closely resemble those of the propionic acid derivatives. It has analgesic and anti-inflammatory properties comparable with those of aspirin, but with a lower incidence of side-effects.

13.1 Absorption, Distribution and Elimination

Azapropazone is well absorbed from the gastrointestinal tract. Food has no effect on absorption. Peak plasma levels are achieved about 4 to 6 hours after a single oral dose and the plasma half-life is relatively long; 12 hours. It is highly protein bound (> 95%). Azapropazone does not undergo extensive biotransformation and is mainly excreted unchanged (about 60 %) in the urine, with the inactive 6-hydroxy metabolite accounting for a further 20 % and 2 to 3 other metabolites of unknown structure for the remainder of the amount measured in the urine. Dosage should therefore be reduced in patients with impaired renal function.

13.2 Drug Interactions

There is not yet adequate evidence to justify the use of azapropazone in patients receiving oral anticoagulants.

13.3 Side-effects

The most common side-effect is gastric intolerance causing nausea or epigastric pain. This is less common than with drugs like aspirin and indomethacin, but may be a little more common than with drugs like ibuprofen. Skin rashes occur occasionally but are mild and respond rapidly to withdrawal of treatment. Despite the chemical similarity of this drug to phenylbutazone, no blood dyscrasias have been reported.

13.4 Clinical Use

Azapropazone is useful in a wide range of rheumatic disorders including rheumatoid arthritis, seronegative arthritis and osteoarthrosis. It has been shown to be as effective as aspirin in rheumatoid arthritis and more effective than ibuprofen in osteoarthrosis. It is probably comparable to naproxen, although direct comparisons have not been made.

13.5 Preparations and Dosage

Azapropazone is available as a 300mg capsule and the usual dosage is 1200mg daily. Doses up to 1800mg daily have been used but the incidence of gastric side-effects is much higher at this level. To date no reports have appeared on its use in childhood.

13.6 Cautions

Azapropazone should be avoided in patients with peptic ulcer until further experience is obtained. It should also be avoided in patients receiving oral anticoagulants until further information has been obtained on this combination of drugs.

14. Diclofenac

Diclofenac is the sodium salt of N-(2-6-dichlorophenyl)-O-aminophenyl acetic acid. It has anti-inflammatory, antipyretic and analgesic actions and also exerts an inhibitory effect on platelet aggregation. It accumulates at sites of inflammation and in low concentrations inhibits prostaglandin synthetase.

14.1 Absorption, Distribution and Metabolism

It is rapidly and completely absorbed by mouth and rectum and is 99 % bound to serum proteins, the presence of high salicylic acid levels diminishing slightly this protein binding. The protein binding is almost entirely to albumin. Its metabolites are largely secreted via the kidney, but partly also in the bile.

14.2 Side-effects

Nausea, vomiting, gastric discomfort and headaches have been reported.

14.3 Clinical Use

Diclofenac has been used in rheumatoid arthritis in children and in adults, in osteoarthrosis, in ankylosing spondylitis and in acute gout. Ghazi and Fowler (1973) observed reduction in swelling of the digits in rheumatoid arthritis and Doreen et al. (1977) noted relief of pain, joint tenderness and swelling and improvement in grip and morning stiffness in rheumatoid arthritis.

14.4 Preparations and Dosage

Tablets of 25mg. Usual daily dosage is 50 to 150mg, in divided doses.

14.5 Cautions

Use with caution in patients with a history of peptic ulceration or dyspepsia.

15. Flurbiprofen

Flurbiprofen is 2-(2-fluoro-4-biphenylyl) propionic acid. It has analgesic and anti-inflammatory properties in animal tests; it is a potent inhibitor of prostaglandin synthetase. The animal tests suggest potent anti-inflammatory activity.

15.1 Absortpion, Distribution and Elimination

Flurbiprofen is well absorbed following oral administration with peak plasma levels achieved 1.5 hours after administration. Absorption bears a linear relationship to dose. It has a relatively short plasma half-life of 3.9 hours. Several metabolites have been identified, but do not seem to contribute to the activity of the drug. Flurbiprofen and its metabolites are excreted in both urine and faeces.

15.2 Drug Interactions

No interactions have been established nor has the safety of the drug when given with other compounds such as oral anticoagulants.

15.3 Side-effects

Flurbiprofen has only recently been introduced and there is to date insufficient experience of its side-effects. It causes less toxic reactions than aspirin; most of those which occur are gastrointestinal but rashes occur occasionally.

15.4 Clinical Use

Flurbiprofen has been shown to be effective in rheumatoid arthritis, osteoarthrosis and ankylosing spondylitis and its effects are comparable with those of full doses of aspirin. Comparisons with other propionic acid derivatives have not yet been reported.

15.5 Preparations and Dosage

Flurbiprofen is available as a 50mg or 100mg tablet. Initial dosage should be 50mg 3 times daily. For pain at night or morning stiffness, the evening dose should be increased to 100mg. Doses up to 300mg daily can be used if the drug proves ineffective at lower dosage.

15.6 Cautions

The drug should not be used in pregnancy, in children or in patients receiving oral anticoagulants, until more is known of its action in these groups of subjects.

References and Recommended Reading

Aspirin

Athreya, B.H.; Moser, G.; Cecil, H.S. and Myers, A.R.: Aspirin-induced hepatotoxicity in juvenile rheumatoid arthritis. A prospective study. Arthritis and Rheumatism 18: 347 (1975).

Boardman, P.L. and Hart, F.D.: Clinical measurement of the anti-inflammatory effects of salicylates in rheumatoid arthritis. British Medical Journal 4: 264 (1967).

Brooks, P.M. and Buchanan, W.W.: in Buchanan and Dick (Eds) Recent Advances in Rheumatology, Part 2 (Churchill Livingstone, Edinburgh 1976).

Cooke, A.R.: Drugs and gastric damage. Drugs 11: 36 (1976).

Graham, G.G.; Champion, G.D.; Day, R.D. and Paull, P.D.: Patterns of plasma concentrations and urinary excretion of salicylate in rheumatoid arthritis. Clinical Pharmacology and Therapeutics 22: 410 (1977).

Klinenberg, J.R. and Miller, R.: Effect of corticosteroids on blood salicylate concentrations. Journal of the American Medical Association 194: 601 (1965).

Lim, R.K.S.: Salicylate analgesia; in Smith and Smith (Eds) The Salicylates: A Critical Bibliographic Review (Wiley, New York 1966).

Mongan, E.; Kelly, P.; Nies, K.; Porter, W.W. and Paulus, H.E.: Tinnitus as an indication of therapeutic serum salicylate levels. Journal of the American Medical Association 226: 142 (1973).

Morley, J.: Proceedings of the Aspirin Symposium, p.19 (Royal College of Surgeons, London 1975).

Muir, A.: in Dixon, Martin, Smith and Wood (Eds) Salicylates, An International Symposium (Little Brown, Boston 1963).

Mustard, J.F. and Packham, M.A.: Factors influencing platelet function: adhesion, release, and aggregation. Pharmacy Revue 22: 97 (1970).

O'Reilly, R.A.: Impact of aspirin and chlorthalidone on the pharmacodynamics of oral anticoagulant drugs in man. Annals of the New York Academy of Science 179: 173 (1971).

Scharrer, I.: Proceedings of the Aspirin Symposium, p.23 (Royal College of Surgeons, London 1975).

Tenney, S.M. and Miller, R.M.: The respiratory and circulatory actions of salicylate. American Journal of Medicine 19: 498 (1955).

Vane, J.R.: in Robinson and Vane (Eds) Prostaglandin Synthetase Inhibitors, p.159 (Raven Press, New York 1974).

Woodbury, D.M. and Fingl, E.: in Goodman and Gilman (Eds) The Pharmacological Basis of Therapeutics, 5th ed, p.328 (Macmillan, New York 1975).

Phenylbutazone

Domenjoz, R.: The pharmacology of phenylbutazone analogues. Annals of the New York Academy of Sciences 86: 263 (1960).

Domenjoz, R.: Synthetic anti-inflammatory drugs: Concepts on their mode of action. Advances in Pharmacology 4: 143 (1966).

Fowler, P.D.: Marrow toxicity of the pyrazoles. Annals of the Rheumatic Diseases 26: 344 (1967).

Fowler, P.D. and Faragher, E.B.: Drug and non-drug factors influencing adverse reactions to pyrazoles. Journal of International Medical Research 5 (Suppl. 2): 108 (1977).

Hart, F.D.: Current therapeutics: Phenylbutazone. Practitioner 171: 84 (1953).

Hansen, J.M. and Christensen, L.K.: Drug interactions with oral sulphonylurea hypoglycaemic drugs. Drugs 13: 24 (1977).

Inman, W.H.: Study of fatal bone marrow depression with special reference to phenylbutazone and oxyphenbutazone. British Medical Journal 1: 1500 (1977).

Koch-Weser, J. and Sellers, E.M.: Drug interactions with coumarin anticoagulants. New England Journal of Medicine 285: 487, 547 (1971).

Kutt, H.: Interactions of antiepileptic drugs. Epilepsia 16: 393 (1975).

Smyth, C.J. and Percy, J.S.: Comparison of indomethacin and phenylbutazone in acute gout. Annals of the Rheumatic Diseases 32: 351 (1973).

Stevenson, A.C.; Bedford, J.; Hill, A.G.S. and Hill, H.F.H.: Chromosomal studies in patients taking phenylbutazone. Annals of the Rheumatic Diseases 30: 487 (1971).

von Rechenberg, H.K.: Phenylbutazone, 2nd ed (Edward Arnold, London 1962).

Walker, S.; Price Evans, D.A.; Benn, P.A.; Littler, T.R. and Halliday, L.D.C.: Phenylbutazone and chromosomal damage. Annals of the Rheumatic Diseases 34: 409 (1975).

Indomethacin

Brooks, P.M.; Bell, M.A.; Sturrock, R.D.; Famaey, J.P. and Dick, W.C.: The clinical significance of indomethacin-probenecid interaction. British Journal of Clinical Pharmacology 1: 287 (1974).

Brooks, P.M.; Walker, J.J.; Bell, M.A.; Buchanan, W.W. and Rhymer, A.R.: Indomethacin-aspirin interaction: a clinical appraisal. British Medical Journal 3: 69 (1975).

Garnham, J.C.; Raymond, K.; Shotton, E. and Turner, P.: The effect of buffered aspirin on plasma indomethacin. European Journal of Clincal Pharmacology 8: 107 (1975).

Hart, F.D. and Boardman, P.L.: Indomethacin: a new non-steroid anti-inflammatory agent. British Medical Journal 2: 965 (1963).

Hart, F.D. and Boardman, P.L.: Indomethacin. Practitioner 192: 828 (1964).

Hart, F.D. and Boardman, P.L.: Indomethacin and phenylbutazone: A comparison. British Medical Journal 2: 1281 (1965).

Lindquist, B.; Moller Jensen, Karen; Johansson, H. and Hansen, T.: Effect of concurrent administration of aspirin and indomethacin on serum concentrations. Clinical Pharamacology and Therapeutics 15: 247 (1974).

Vessel, E.S.; Passananti, G.T. and Johnson, Alice O.: Failure of indomethacin and warfarin to interact in normal human volunteers. Journal of Clinical Pharamacology 15: 486 (1975).

Ibuprofen

Davies, E.F. and Avery, G.S: Ibuprofen: A review of its pharmacological properties and therapeutic efficacy in rheumatic disorders. Drugs 2: 416 (1971).

Huskisson, E.C.; Woolf, D.L.; Balme, H.W.; Scott, Jane and Franklyn, Sue: Four new anti-inflammatory drugs: responses and variations. British Medical Journal 1: 1048 (1976).

Naproxen

Brogden, R.N.; Pinder, R.M.; Sawyer, Phyllis R.; Speight, T.M. and Avery, G.S.: Naproxen: A review of its pharmacological properties and therapeutic efficacy and use. Drugs 9: 326 (1975).

Hart, F.D. and Matts, S.G.F.: Naproxen (Naprosyn) and gastrointestinal haemorrhage. British Medical Journal 2: 51 (1974).

Hill, H.F.; Hill, A.G.; Mowat, A.G.; Ansell, B.M.; Mathews, J.A.; Seifert, M.H.; Gumpel, J.M. and Christie, G.A.: Naproxen. A new non-hormonal anti-inflammatory agent. Studies in rheumatoid arthritis. Annals of the Rheumatic Diseases 33: 12 (1974).

Huskisson, E.C.; Woolf, D.L.; Balme, H.W.; Scott, Jane and Franklyn, Sue: Four new anti-inflammatory drugs: responses and variations. British Medical Journal 1: 1048 (1976).

Roth, S.H. and Boost, G.: An open trial of naproxen in rheumatoid arthritis patients with significant esophageal, gastric and duodenal lesions. Journal of Clinical Pharmacology 15: 378 (1975).

Segre, E.J.: Naproxen metabolism in man. Journal of Clinical Pharmacology 15: 316 (1975).

Fenoprofen

Brogden, R.N.; Pinder, R.M.; Speight, T.M. and Avery, G.S.: Fenoprofen: A review of its pharmacological properties and therapeutic efficacy in rheumatic diseases. Drugs 13: 241 (1977).

Gruber, C.M. Jr.: Clinical pharmacology of fenoprofen: a review. Journal of Rheumatology 3 (Suppl 2): 8 (1976).

Huskisson, E.C.; Wojtulewski, J.A.; Berry, H.; Scott, Jane; Hart, F.D. and Balme, H.W.: Treatment of rheumatoid arthritis with fenoprofen. Comparison with aspirin. British Medical Journal 1: 176 (1974).

Huskisson, E.C.; Woolf, D.L.; Balme, H.W.; Scott, Jane and Franklyn, Sue: Four new anti-inflammatory drugs: responses and variations. British Medical Journal 1: 1048 (1976).

Ketoprofen

Huskisson, E.C.; Wolf, D.L.; Balme, H.W.; Scott, Jane and Franklyn, Sue: Four new anti-inflammatory drugs: responses and variations. British Medical Journal 1: 1048 (1976).

Alclofenac

Aylward, M.; Parker, R.J.; Holly, F.; Maddock, J. and Davies, D.A.S.: Long-term study of indomethacin and alclofenac in treatment of rheumatoid arthritis. British Medical Journal 2: 7 (1975).

Billings, R.A.; Burry, H.C.; Emslie, F.S. and Kerr, G.D: Vasculitis with alclofenac therapy. British Medical Journal 4: 263 (1974).

Brogden, R.N.; Heel, R.C.; Speight, T.M. and Avery, G.S.: Alclofenac: A review of its pharmacological properties and therapeutic efficacy in rheumatoid arthritis and allied rheumatic disorders. Drugs 14: 241 (1977).

Hort, J.F.: Adverse reactions to alclofenac. Current Medical Research and Opinion 3: 333 (1975).

Tolmetin

Ehrlich, G.E. and Roth, S.: Rheumatoid arthritis: long-term therapy with tolmetin sodium. Orthopaedics Digest 4: 16 (1976).

Huskisson, E.C.; Berry, H.; Scott, J. and Balme, H.W.: Tolectin for rheumatoid arthritis. Rheumatology and Rehabilitation 13: 132 (1974).

Selley, M.L.; Glass, J.; Triggs, E.J. and Thomas, J.: Pharmacokinetic studies of tolmetin in man. Clinical Pharmacology and Therapeutics 17: 599 (1975).

Sulindac

Duggan, D.E.; Hare, L.E.; Ditzler, C.A.; Lei, B.W. and Kwan, K.C.: The disposition of sulindac. Clinical Pharmacology and Therapeutics 21: 326 (1977).

Huskisson, E.C. and Franchimont, P.: Clinoril in the Treatment of Rheumatic Disorders (Raven Press, New York 1976).

Various Authors: Special symposium on sulindac. Worldwide perspective. European Journal of Rheumatology and Inflammation 1: 6-68 (1978).

Flufenamic Acid

Brooks, P.M. and Buchanan, W.W.: in Buchanan and Dick (Eds) Recent Advances in Rheumatology, Part 2, p.54 (Churchill Livingstone, Edinburgh 1976).

Holmes, E.L.: Fenemates in medicine. Annals of Physical Medicine 36: Suppl. (1967).

Azapropazone

Grennan, D.M.; Watkins, C. and Kennedy, A.C.: Preliminary clinical evaluation of azapropazone in rheumatoid arthritis. Current Medical Research and Opinion 2: 67 (1974).

Various Authors: Recent advances in clinical rheumatology: A review and clinical assessment of azapropazone. Current Medical Research and Opinion 4: 3-100 (1976).

Diclofenac

Doreen, M.S.; Boardman, P.L.; Fowler, P.D. and Poole, P.H.: Diclofenac in rheumatoid arthritis. Rheumatism and Rehabilitation. In press (1977).

Ghazi, S.A. and Fowler, P.D.: A clinical trial of a new anti-inflammatory analgesic compound in rheumatoid arthritis. Journal of International Medical Research 1: 591 (1973).

Krupp, P.J.; Menasse-Gdynia, R.; Sallman, A.; Wilhelmi, G.; Ziel, R. and Jaques, R.: Sodium O-[2,6-dichlorophenyl)-amino]-phenyl -acetate(GP 45,840), a new non-steroidal anti-inflammatory agent. Experientia (Basle) 29: 450 (1973).

Ku, E.C.; Wasvary, J.M. and Cash, W.D.: Diclofenac sodium 450 (GP 45,840) a potent inhibitor of prostaglandin synthetase. Biochemical Pharmacology 24: 641 (1975).

Flurbiprofen

Various Authors: Symposium on Froben. Current Medical Research and Opinion 3 (Suppl. 4) (1975).

Chapter III

Drugs Which Apparently Affect the Rheumatoid Disease Process ('long-term or specific' agents)

In the 1920's, the many similar clinical features of tuberculous disease and rheumatoid arthritis made some clinicians of the time feel that there might be some connection between the two conditions. In both diseases, fever, anaemia, systemic upset and wasting occurred and in many cases of tuberculous disease the tubercle bacillus could not be isolated. On these slender grounds, as gold salts had been used in the treatment of pulmonary tuberculosis, particularly by Holger Mollgaard in Denmark, it was tried entirely empirically in rheumatoid arthritis. It was Jacques Forestier's clinical studies however, that led to its introduction as a regular and orthodox form of therapy for rheumatoid arthritis; for, although its mode of action is still uncertain, it appears to lead to remission or resolution of the disease in many cases.

On equally slender and highly empirical grounds, d-penicillamine, the anti-malarials chloroquine and hydroxychloroquine and the so-called immunosuppressive or cytotoxic agents have also been similarly used, often successfully, but at the expense of not infrequent and occasionally serious side-effects. All these agents take several weeks to produce relief and if later they are prematurely stopped relapse is delayed by a similar but rather shorter period. Clearly, the mode of action of these drugs is entirely different from that seen with the more rapidly acting agents such as aspirin, indomethacin or corticosteroids.

Correct use of these 'long-term specific' agents is in patients with acute inflammatory rheumatoid changes with active progressive and erosive disease (when anti-inflammatory analgesics only provide symptomatic relief), not in chronic and advanced destructive disease. With all these agents prolonged therapy is essential: if remission is induced prolonged maintenance suppressive therapy for many months or, usually, years is essential to maintain that improvement.

All these agents are potentially toxic, sometimes seriously so, and before embarking on such a long-term course of treatment the same full consultation and discussion with patient, relatives and general medical attendant is called for as would take place before any serious major surgical operation. Long-term courses with any of these agents should only be undertaken by physicians with full laboratory facilities, and, in the case of the antimalarials, the assistance of an ophthalmological colleague.

Since with all these long-term agents some weeks may elapse before any clinical effect becomes apparent, quick acting anti-inflammatory agents have to be used concurrently, initially in all, and additionally throughout the period of therapy in many cases. This combination of slow and quick acting agents is necessary in most cases, but it is wise to avoid giving two agents which may have similar side-effects (e.g. gold salts and phenylbutazone).

1. Gold

Gold salts are the oldest member of the group of 'specific' drugs for long-term use in rheumatoid arthritis. That they have survived since their introduction in the 1920's is tribute to their effectiveness. However, only in the last 10 years has the correct way of using gold become apparent. The mode of action of gold is unknown.

1.1 Absorption, Distribution and Elimination

Sodium aurothiomalate (gold sodium thiomalate) is rapidly absorbed from the site of intramuscular injection and peak plasma levels of 400 to 700μg/100ml are achieved within 2 to 6 hours of injection. It has a long half-life of 5 to 6 days so that the plasma level has declined to about half of its peak level after a week, when the next dose is given. After a few weeks of regular injections, a steady state is achieved. The exact mode of excretion is not known but gold is found in both urine and faeces. It is taken up by macrophages and is identifiable in the reticuloendothelial system and in synovium, where it remains for long periods of time.

There is a wide individual variation in plasma levels achieved during gold therapy but there is no convincing evidence that this is related to the patient's response. It has been suggested that plasma gold levels might be a more logical way of controlling therapy (Lorber, 1977; Lorber et al., 1973) but the lack of consistent direct correlation between plasma levels and response does not support this. In practice, clinical effects seem to be the best guide to therapy. Gold plasma levels are not related to the toxic effects of the drug and are not of value in predicting their development.

1.2. Drug Interactions

It is unwise to give gold with other drugs which may affect the bone marrow such as immunosuppressives, penicillamine or phenylbutazone, although there is no direct evidence that this is harmful.

1.3 Side-effects

Gold has three major side-effects, blood dyscrasias, proteinuria and rashes. These are important because they are dangerous to life and because they prevent the continuation of gold therapy in many patients. Gold is one of the more potentially dangerous drugs, deaths resulting from aplastic anaemia, haemorrhage from thrombbocytopenia, or, more rarely, from agranulocytosis.

The most common side-effect is a rash, which occurs most often after a few months of treatment and develops in about 30% of patients treated. Rashes are of variable severity, sometimes mild and rapidly resolving, sometimes severe, even exfoliative, and lasting for as long as a year. Although some clinicians suggest using small doses of gold after the rash has resolved, it often recurs and the further use of gold is hazardous.

Proteinuria and nephrotic syndrome probably occur with about the same frequency as in patients on penicillamine. As with penicillamine, biopsy shows the presence of immune complex deposition and the condition resolves slowly upon withdrawal of treatment.

Agranulocytosis and aplastic anaemia may develop at any time during the course of treatment with gold. The exact incidence is not clear but these reactions are rare. Thrombocytopenia is not uncommon. Because of this risk, full blood and platelet counts must be carried out at least monthly in patients on gold.

Mouth ulcers may occur with or without a rash in patients receiving gold. Hypersensitivity reactions may occur and it is wise to give a small test dose of 10mg before proceeding with further doses.

1.4 Clinical Use

Gold is effective in rheumatoid arthritis, producing a response in about 80% of patients. It acts in seronegative as well as seropositive patients and exerts its principal effect on the active synovitis of the disease. Joint swelling declines; pain and stiffness are reduced. This effect is achieved slowly. Most patients begin to respond after 4 to 16 weeks of treatment and the maximum effect of the drug is seen after 3 to 6 months. As with penicillamine, there is a reduction in the number and size of nodules and in some other extra-articular features of the disease. There is a reduction in the requirements for other drugs, including corticosteroids. Rheumatoid factor titre and ESR fall but these laboratory changes are not a good guide to the response of an individual patient.

Gold is an alternative to penicillamine in patients with persistently active or progressive disease and should be used early in the course of the disease before irreversible anatomical changes have developed. There is a relationship between response to gold and response to penicillamine, so that patients who respond to one are likely to respond to the other and patients who fail to respond to one, often but not always, fail to respond to the other. Gold has been shown to have a small effect on delaying the progression of X-ray changes in one study (Sigler et al., 1974), but in this respect it is less effective than penicillamine or azathioprine. Clinical changes are similar with these three drugs but gold is more often withdrawn than penicillamine because of toxicity. This is a disadvantage since these treatments are used to control the disease and it is essential to continue treatment for long periods of time.

Gold is also effective in palindromic rheumatism and in juvenile chronic polyarthritis, especially the juvenile rheumatoid arthritis variety. About 60 % of children respond (see chapt. XIX; sect. 4.2).

1.5 Preparations and Dosage

Gold salts are given by intramuscular injection. Using sodium aurothiomalate, a test dose of 10mg is given followed by 50mg at weekly intervals. Once a response is obtained, the interval between injections is increased at first to 2, then to 4 or 6 weeks and the drug is continued indefinitely. The concept of a 1g course of gold is out of date and should be discarded. It has no scientific basis. Maintenance doses are required to prevent relapse and this is particularly important since second courses are usually ineffective. At the first sign of a relapse in a patient on maintenance doses, the interval between injections should be reduced until the disease is again controlled. Patients who have failed to respond after 4 months of gold therapy may be given 100mg weekly for a few weeks when a few more may respond. After this time, response is unlikely.

Another preparation, the thioglucose, is available in some countries (Rothermich et al., 1976). It is equally effective and may have a lower tendency to cause side-effects.

1.6 Cautions

It is unwise to give gold with other drugs which suppress the bone marrow. Monthly blood counts and weekly urinalysis are required during treatment and patients should be warned to report any possible adverse reactions to their physician. The results of the last urine tests and blood counts must always be known before the next injection is given. Gold therapy should be avoided in pregnancy.

2. D-Penicillamine

D-Penicillamine is β,β-dimethylcysteine, a degradation product of penicillin. It is one of a group of drugs which can be said to have a 'specific' long-term action in rheumatoid arthritis. Its action is slow, and selective since it does not benefit all types of inflammatory arthritis. It exerts its effects on extra-articular features of the disease as well as on joints, and there is reduction in rheumatoid factor and ESR. In patients able to continue treatment, there is improvement in the outcome of the disease as judged by delay in radiological progression. The mode of action of the drug is unknown. It was first used because of its ability to reduce titres of circulating rheumatoid factor (Jaffe, 1970), but this is almost certainly not its mode of action.

2.1 Absorption and Elimination

No method exists for measuring penicillamine blood levels and there is little knowledge of its absorption or excretion, but it seems that there is some hepatic metabolism and rapid renal excretion of unchanged drug. Certainly, the effects on the disease are not clearly related to the presence of circulating penicillamine which has an immediate effect on rheumatoid factor.

2.2. Drug Interactions

Penicillamine can safely be given with other analgesic and anti-inflammatory drugs, including corticosteroids but it is probably wise to avoid using it with phenylbutazone as both drugs affect the bone marrow. The combination of penicillamine and azathioprine is particularly likely to cause marrow aplasia.

2.3 Side-effects

The side-effects of penicillamine are shown in table I, with their approximate frequency and time of onset. Knowledge of the side-effects of the drug and their management is essential if patients are to be looked after safely and treatment continued. Side-effects tend to occur at particular times during the course of treatment, so that surveillance should be planned to detect side-effects at certain times. The overall incidence of side-effects is greatest in the first few months and problems are infrequent after 18 months of treatment.

Nausea and anorexia are among the earliest problems, developing within the first few weeks of treatment. The incidence is greatly reduced by using a gradually increasing dose. Occasional patients develop intractable vomiting and have to stop treatment but in most cases, nausea and anorexia are transient and do not interfere with treatment.

Impairment or loss of taste may develop after about 6 weeks of treatment. It is wise to warn patients of this possibility and advise them of its outcome. Taste returns after about 6 weeks whether the drug is continued or not, so that it is pointless to interrupt treatment. Copper salts do not prevent the complication and have no place in its treatment.

Rashes developing during penicillamine therapy are of two main types. One is an early rash which develops within the first few months of treatment. It is an 'allergic'

Table I. Side-effects of penicillamine and approximate frequency

Effect	Incidence	Onset
Nausea, anorexia	25%	First few weeks
Rash	25%	Early onset (first few months) and late onset (after 6 months or more)
Loss of taste	25%	About 6 weeks
Thrombocytopenia	15%	Any time
Proteinuria	15%	After 4 or more months
Nephrotic syndrome	5%	Within weeks of developing proteinuria
Mouth ulceration	5%	
Neutropenia	rare	Any time
Febrile reactions	rare	First few doses
Systemic lupus erythematosus	rare	After 1 or 2 years
Myasthenia gravis	rare	After 1 to 2 years
Joint creaking or pain	rare	Anytime
Goodpasture syndrome	rare	After 1 to 2 years

type of rash, maculopapular, and resembles that produced by ampicillin. It disappears within days of stopping treatment and does not usually recur when the drug is restarted at a low dose and gradually increased. The other type is a late rash, which is a much bigger problem although it is fortunately less common. It develops after 6 months of treatment or more. The lesions are raised irregular plaques with scaly surfaces, very itchy and unresponsive to treatment with topical corticosteroids. This rash disappears slowly when the drug is withdrawn but often recurs when it is restarted. Less common rashes which may occur in patients receiving penicillamine include elastosis perforans serpiginosa, epidermolysis bullosa, pemphigus, urticaria, and those occurring with other features of systemic lupus erythematosus.

Proteinuria is one of the more important complications of penicillamine because it may lead to withdrawal of treatment. It develops after 4 or more months of treatment and is of variable severity. Between a quarter and a third of all patients who develop proteinuria become nephrotic and this usually happens within weeks of the development of proteinuria. Renal biopsy in patients with proteinuria shows the presence of immune complexes in most cases. Whether the treatment is stopped or not, the proteinuria gradually diminishes but often takes a year or more to disappear. It is not necessary to stop treatment in patients with less than 5g daily of proteinuria who do not become nephrotic but a close watch should be kept on their renal function. The greatest hazard of this complication is in patients with pre-existing renal disease; the elderly, for example, in whom reduction in blood volume leads to uraemia.

Thrombocytopenia is the most common haematological disorder in patients receiving penicillamine. Unfortunately it is unpredictable and occurs at any time during the course of treatment. Suppression to less than 150,000 platelets per cu mm occurs in about 15% of patients, but serious suppression to less than 50,000 per cu mm occurs much less often, in about 5% of patients. Bleeding episodes are even more unusual. When thrombocytopenia occurs, the drug should be stopped and rapid recovery is usual. It can usually be cautiously restarted and providing that the doses are kept down, safely continued.

Neutropenia is much less common and much more serious. There appears to be a really serious variety of blood dyscrasia which is quite different from the transient thrombocytopenia. In such patients, levels of white cells and platelets continue to fall after the drug has been stopped and bone marrow shows absence of precursors. Recovery may occur but a few deaths have been reported.

Mouth ulcers are occasionally a problem in patients on penicillamine and, if severe, may lead to withdrawal of treatment. Local corticosteroid therapy may help.

Febrile reactions occasionally occur after the first few tablets of penicillamine. These patients sometimes seem to be very sensitive to the drug and may respond well to very small doses.

Systemic lupus erythematosus is a rare and late complication, developing after 1 or 2 years of treatment. Arthralgia and rashes appear to be the most common manifestations and patients may note that the joint pain is quite different from their original arthritis. Antinuclear factor is strongly positive, LE cells may be present and antibodies to DNA have been described in such cases. The disease disappears when the drug is stopped.

A few fatal cases of a Goodpasture-like syndrome have been reported and a few cases of myasthenia gravis, responding to withdrawal of penicillamine.

One of the most difficult problems in patients receiving penicillamine is an exacerbation of arthritis in a patient who was previously well controlled. Cases of joint pain and creaking have been reported which respond to reduction in dosage. Another possible cause is drug-induced systemic lupus erythematosus. It seems that some patients continue to have exacerbations of disease but at a much lower level than before treatment with penicillamine and it is often worth waiting for a few months to see if remission will follow relapse. Occasional patients seem to escape from control by the drug and it is necessary to stop treatment and seek an alternative.

2.4 Clinical Use

Penicillamine is effective in rheumatoid arthritis, producing a reasonable response in about 80% of patients. The remaining 20% do not benefit. Amongst these patients is an excess of those with severe destructive disease of weight-bearing joints, but sometimes an apparently highly suitable patient with early active disease just fails to respond. Seronegative patients do just as well as those who are seropositive. The principal effect of the drug is on active synovitis which is controlled. Active inflammation and proliferation of synovial tissues disappears in patients who do well. This effect is achieved slowly, the greatest effect of the drug being seen in the second month of treatment and the maximum effect after 4 to 6 months. There is a reduction in the number and size of rheumatoid nodules, improvement in tenosynovitis, extensor sheath swellings and lymphadenopathy and sometimes in peripheral neuropathy, splenomegaly and leg ulcers.

Penicillamine is probably the most useful drug for patients with vasculitis but although dramatic results have been reported in some cases of peripheral gangrene, not all patients benefit. Penicillamine therapy leads to a reduction in the requirements for other drugs, including corticosteroids.

The correct use of penicillamine is for patients with persistently active or progressive disease. It should seldom be used in the first 6 months of the disease because spontaneous improvement is common at this stage. Nor should the start of treatment be delayed much after 6 months because complete recovery is impossible once permanent anatomical changes have developed. Penicillamine therapy is unlikely to help in patients whose symptoms are due to mechanical problems such as atlanto-axial subluxation.

Penicillamine is as effective as gold and azathioprine. Although it causes more side-effects than gold, it is less likely to be withdrawn than gold and has a greater suppressive effect on radiological changes. For these reasons, it now represents the first choice of drugs of this group. It is more effective than anti-inflammatory therapy, including corticosteroids.

Penicillamine is also effective in about 50% of cases of juvenile chronic polyarthritis, particularly those with juvenile rheumatoid arthritis. It is useful in palindromic rheumatism but it has not been shown to be helpful in any other type of arthritis.

2.5 Preparations and Dosage

Penicillamine is available as 50, 125 or 250mg tablets. In adults with chronic rheumatoid arthritis, it should be started at a dose of 125 to 250mg daily and this is increased by 125 to 250mg daily at intervals of 2 to 8 weeks depending on the urgency of treatment. If side-effects such as nausea develop, no further increase in dosage is made until the problem has resolved. Similarly, once patients start to improve, no further increase in dosage is made. The usual maintenance dose is 500mg to 1g daily. Occasional patients require less and a few require more. In palindromic rheumatism, a dose of 250mg daily is often sufficient. In juvenile chronic polyarthritis, the initial daily dose is 50mg increasing to between 250mg and 600mg, depending on the patients size.

2.6 Cautions

Serious consideration should be given before penicillamine is given to patients with renal disease because of the danger of superimposed nephrotic syndrome and reduction of glomerular filtration rate. Patients receiving penicillamine should be seen at least monthly, with urinalysis and a full blood count including platelets carried out every 3 to 4 weeks. Patients should also be warned to report any unexpected reactions to the physician who is supervising the treatment.

The use of penicillamine should be avoided in pregnancy, although a number of normal pregnancies have been reported in treated patients with conditions other than rheumatoid arthritis.

3. Azathioprine

Azathioprine is 6-(1-methyl-4-nitro imidazol-5-yl-thio) purine. It is an anti-metabolite which acts by interfering with purine biosynthesis. Its action in rheumatoid arthritis is presumed to arise from its immunosuppressive effect. It is the first choice of immunosuppressive for use in rheumatoid arthritis because it is less toxic and easier to use than alternative drugs such as cyclophosphamide or methotrexate.

3.1 Absorption and Elimination

Azathioprine is well absorbed when given by mouth and has a plasma half-life of about 3 hours. It is first converted in the body to 6-mercaptopurine and then to thiouric acid by the enzyme xanthine oxidase and excreted either in this form, or in large part (50%) as unchanged 6-mercaptopurine. Dosage of azathioprine must therefore be reduced in patients with renal failure.

3.2 Drug Interactions

Because allopurinol inhibits the enzyme xanthine oxidase, it interferes with the metabolic degradation of 6-mercaptopurine formed from azathioprine and enhances the toxicity of the drug. Azathioprine must be given in reduced dosage (to about 25% of usual) in patients receiving allopurinol. Azathioprine should not be used with penicillamine or other drugs which may produce marrow toxicity.

3.3 Side-effects

The most important toxic reactions are marrow suppression, gastrointestinal intolerance and infections. Leucopenia is the most common haematological problem but thrombocytopenia or pancytopenia may occur. Regular blood counts are essential and the drug should be stopped if serious suppression occurs. In most cases this is dose-related and the drug can be restarted at a lower dose.

Nausea, vomiting and diarrhoea occur in about 15 % of patients, usually within days or weeks of starting treatment. In many cases, the drug must be stopped but it is sometimes possible to treat it with symptomatic remedies.

Infections include herpes zoster, warts and sometimes more serious infections such as recurrent pneumonia. Opportunistic infections with unusual organisms or fungi may occur and should be considered in patients who become ill during treatment.

There is an increased incidence of malignancy in patients receiving azathioprine following renal transplantation and malignancies have been reported occasionally in rheumatic patients. An increased incidence of malignancy has not yet been established in rheumatoid arthritis and it does not appear to be a significant hazard on present evidence. Occasional side-effects include rash, drug fever and other hypersensitivity reactions and alopecia. Chromosomal abnormalities have been reported but are of doubtful clinical significance. Azoospermia does not occur.

3.4 Clinical Use

The action of azathioprine in rheumatoid arthritis resembles that of penicillamine and gold. There is a gradual suppression of disease activity with relief of pain, reduction in joint swelling and other signs of inflammation. Maximum effectiveness is achieved after 4 to 6 months of treatment and ESR and rheumatoid factor titres fall. There is slowing of radiological progression and it is possible to reduce the doses of other drugs, including corticosteroids. Azathioprine is effective in about 80 % of patients treated, either seronegative and seropositive, but, as with other drugs of this type, results are unpredictable.

The clinical effects of azathioprine are similar to those of gold and penicillamine but azathioprine is superior to gold in its effect on slowing radiological progression of the disease. It is probably a little less effective than cyclophosphamide but certainly less toxic.

Azathioprine is used in rheumatoid arthritis as an alternative to gold and penicillamine, for patients with persistently active or progressive disease. Since response probably does not have any relationship with response to penicillamine and gold, it is a useful drug for patients who fail to respond to either penicillamine or gold. It is also useful for difficult cases of psoriatic arthropathy which fail to respond to non-steroidal anti-inflammatory analgesics. It is used in systemic lupus erythematosus, particularly for patients who require excessive doses of corticosteroids to control the disease. It is effective in Wegener's granulomatosis and is sometimes used in cases of polymyositis which fail to respond well to corticosteroids.

3.5 Preparations and Dosage

Azathioprine is available as a 50mg tablet and the usual dosage is 150mg daily in 2 or 3 divided doses, or 2.5mg per kg per day. Trials however, have shown that smaller doses are equally effective in rheumatoid arthritis and it seems sensible to give 100mg daily for the first few months, increasing only if the response is unsatisfactory.

3.6 Cautions

Full blood counts are required at least monthly in patients receiving azathioprine. The dose should be reduced to 25% of usual in patients on allopurinol. Other drugs which suppress the bone marrow should not be used.

Azathioprine should be used seldom and only if there are most pressing indications in young adults because of the possible effects that azathioprine might have on their offspring. It should be avoided in pregnancy and in children.

4. Chloroquine and Hydroxychloroquine

Chloroquine and hydroxychloroquine, 4-aminoquinoline compounds, are antimalarials which are also occasionally used for the long-term treatment of rheumatoid arthritis and systemic lupus erythematosus. In rheumatoid arthritis they have a slow delayed therapeutic action resembling that of gold salts. Their use is limited by ocular toxicity.

4.1 Absorption, Distribution and Elimination

Chloroquine and hydroxychloroquine behave similarly. They are well absorbed from the gastrointestinal tract. Steady-state plasma levels of chloroquine are reached after about 10 days of regular dosing and the drug has a long plasma half-life of about 6 days. Chloroquine is mainly excreted unchanged in the urine (70%) but a small part is metabolised. Excretion occurs to some extent by non-renal mechanisms in renal failure but dosage should be modified for prolonged treatment in those with severely impaired renal function. Chloroquine is concentrated in liver, spleen, kidney, lung, central nervous system and white blood cells within the body. When the drug is stopped, it may take months or years for the remaining drug to be excreted.

4.2 Side-effects

The most important adverse reaction is retinopathy which occurs in about 10% of patients treated with 250mg per day or more of chloroquine for at least 1 year.

Once symptoms of impaired vision have become apparent, the defect is irreversible and may progress to blindness even if the drug is stopped. It is therefore essential to make regular ophthalmic examinations and to stop the drug at the first sign of visual impairment; certainly before the patient notices any visual changes. This complication seems to be dose-related and can be avoided by using low-dose or intermittent therapy. There is destruction of the retina with pigmentation and arterial constriction. Reversible corneal opacities and field defects may also occur.

Apart from eye changes, chloroquine is usually well tolerated; in fact it is probably the best tolerated of the drugs with this 'specific' type of action. Nausea, vomiting, pruritus, rashes and depigmentation and loss of hair occur occasionally. Fetal abnormalities have been reported (Hart and Naunton, 1964) and the drug should not be given in pregnancy.

4.3 Clinical Use

In rheumatoid arthritis, chloroquine has an action resembling that of gold and clinical trials have shown that these two drugs are equally effective. There is a slow improvement in symptoms and signs which develops over the course of a few months treatment. There is improvement in extra-articular features of the disease, and reduction in ESR and rheumatoid factor titre, but there is no evidence for any slowing down of radiological progression of the disease. Chloroquine is therefore an alternative to gold, penicillamine and immunosuppressives. Most clinicians prefer these compounds, fearing the ocular toxicity of chloroquine, but chloroquine still has some supporters who would use it before the other drugs.

Indications for use are the same as for gold and penicillamine; persistently active disease despite optimum anti-inflammatory therapy, and, progressive disease. Like other drugs of this type, there is little point in short courses of treatment. If the drug is to be used at all, it is to control the disease and this inevitably demands long-term treatment, but it is in these long-term cases that eye changes are a particular hazard, so that many clinicians prefer to discontinue therapy after 12 or 18 months. It seems that retinal damage is more likely to occur if therapy is continued daily for longer than a year or if total dosage has exceeded 1.6g/kg body weight.

Chloroquine is sometimes useful in the milder cases of systemic lupus erythematosus and especially in those with troublesome chronic skin lesions. It is occasionally used in juvenile chronic arthritis as an alternative to gold salts (Laaksonen et al., 1974). It should not be used in psoriatic arthropathy since the skin lesions may be exacerbated.

4.4 Dosage and Preparations

One may use chloroquine phosphate (250mg tablet; 155mg base), chloroquine sulphate (200mg tablet; 150mg base), or hydroxychloroquine sulphate (200mg tablet;

156mg base). Usual dosages for adults with rheumatoid arthritis are 200 or 250mg daily for chloroquine sulphate or phosphate and 400 to 600mg daily for hydroxychloroquine sulphate. It is wise to start with a low dose, increasing after 3 months in the absence of an adequate response. In children, the dosage of chloroquine is 3mg/kg/day and of hydroxychloroquine 5mg/kg/day.

4.5 Cautions

Ophthalmic examination including examination of visual fields with red and white light should be carried out before the start of treatment, carefully documented and repeated every 3 months. The drug should be stopped at the first sign of ocular toxicity. Some clinicians prefer to stop treatment for a time after 1 or 2 years. Patients should be warned of the possibility of visual changes and advised to report at once if this occurs.

Chloroquine should not be given with phenylbutazone, gold salts, penicillamine or immunosuppressive drugs. A full blood count should be carried out every 6 months, although blood dyscrasias are unusual.

Chloroquine should never be given in pregnancy, to patients with visual abnormalities or to patients with psoriasis, in whom the skin lesions may be exacerbated.

5. Cyclophosphamide

Cyclophosphamide is 2(di-(2-chlorethyl)-amino)-1-oxa-3 aza-2-phosphacyclohexane 2-oxide monohydrate. It is an alkylating agent which is believed to be effective in rheumatoid arthritis and other rheumatic disorders because of its immunosuppressive effect. Like azathioprine it has a slow onset of action and causes improvement in extra-articular as well as articular features. It may also be useful in some other diseases, such as systemic lupus erythematosus, but because of its serious side-effects it is not recommended in non-malignant conditions. *Thus, in rheumatic disorders cyclophosphamide is best reserved for very serious cases likely to prove fatal and who have failed to respond to other 'specific' agents.*

5.1 Absorption, Distribution and Elimination

Cyclophosphamide is well absorbed from the gut. Peak blood levels are achieved within an hour of administration and it has a plasma half-life of 4 to 6.5 hours. It is not or only slightly bound to plasma proteins (0 to 10%), although its active metabolites are more protein bound (56%). It is excreted in urine and faeces either as unchanged drug or metabolites, some with alkylating activity. The drug must be activated before it becomes effective and this takes place in the liver.

5.2 Drug Interactions

Drugs which increase liver microsomal drug metabolising enzyme activity, such as barbiturates, may increase both the effectiveness and toxicity of cyclophosphamide by stimulating its activation in the liver (see above). Drugs which decrease liver microsomal enzyme activity such as phenothiazines may reduce its effectiveness by inhibiting its activation in the liver. Such combinations should be avoided and it is also wise to avoid other drugs which may suppress the bone marrow, including gold and phenylbutazone. Allopurinol also increases the risk of bone marrow depression in patients concurrently treated with cyclophosphamide (see chapt. VII; sect. 4.3).

5.3 Side-effects and Toxicity

The principal side-effects are nausea, vomiting and diarrhoea, bone marrow suppression, stomatitis, haemorrhagic cystitis, infections, alopecia and infertility. Cyclophosphamide is a very toxic drug.

Bone marrow suppression is a direct effect and is dose-related. A careful watch must be kept on haemoglobin, white count and platelets during treatment. Suppression of neutrophil count is the most common problem and this usually responds rapidly to withdrawal of treatment. The drug can then be reintroduced at a lower dose.

Gastrointestinal side-effects are an early problem which occasionally limit the use of the drug, as may stomatitis.

Haemorrhagic cystitis is a potentially serious side-effect and demands immediate withdrawal of the drug. Some patients have dysuria which may require reduction in dosage. Bladder fibrosis may occur after several years of treatment and bladder carcinoma has been reported.

Alopecia occurs in about 20% of patients receiving 100mg daily and may be total. The hair regrows slowly if the drug is stopped. Patients should be warned in advance of this possibility.

Infections presumably arise because of the drug's immunosuppressive action. They vary from herpes zoster to more serious opportunistic infections with unusual organisms. This is a particular hazard which should be considered in any patient with rheumatoid arthritis.

Azoospermia or amenorrhoea are common in patients receiving cyclophosphamide and infertility is therefore also usual.

Hepatotoxicity may occur with raised enzyme levels and liver function tests should be checked from time to time.

There is a suspicion that treatment with cyclophosphamide might lead to an increase in the incidence of malignancy, although no such increase has yet been shown in patients with rheumatic disorders. Because of the risk of dysmorphogenic effects, the drug should be avoided in pregnancy and in patients of either sex who may contribute to child-bearing. As stated above, because of its toxic potential, cyclophosphamide should be reserved for very serious cases.

5.4 Clinical Use

Despite its toxicity, cyclophosphamide is undoubtedly highly effective in rheumatoid arthritis. It has a similar type of action to drugs such as penicillamine and gold. It works slowly and the effect on joints is accompanied by changes in extra-articular features of the disease. ESR and rheumatoid factor titres are reduced. It has a potent effect on the progression of X-ray changes. It is probably a little more effective than gold and certainly it is more effective in preventing radiological progression. Withdrawal of treatment is necessary in about 50% of patients, rather more than with gold and a little more common than in patients receiving azathioprine. Toxicity is the usual reason for stopping treatment. Because of its toxicity, cyclophosphamide should be reserved for the most desperate cases. It is the last resort in patients who have failed to respond to drugs like gold, penicillamine and azathioprine and in those with life threatening complications. In this situation, chlorambucil may be preferable because it has less side-effects (see section 6).

Cyclophosphamide is also used in severe cases of systemic lupus erythematosus (see chapter XIII) and occasionally in some rare rheumatic diseases such as Wegener's granulomatosis. It has a potent steroid-sparing effect which is useful in any condition when corticosteroid requirements are excessive.

5.5 Preparations and Dosage

Cyclophosphamide is available as a 50mg tablet. Dosage should be kept to a minimum since many side-effects are dose-related. The range of dosage is 1.0 to 1.5mg/kg per day in divided doses and most patients with rheumatoid arthritis require 50 to 100mg daily. Patients should be started on 50mg daily and dosage increased no more often than monthly.

5.6 Cautions

Cyclophosphamide should be avoided in the reproductive age group, in children and in pregnancy. The most pressing indications are required to justify using the drug in these circumstances. No other drug which may suppress the bone marrow should be given concurrently. Blood counts should be carried out at least monthly and patients warned to report at once if serious side-effects develop.

6. Chlorambucil

Chlorambucil is p-(di-2-chloroethyl) aminophenyl butyric acid. Like cyclophosphamide it is an alkylating agent which has been used in the treatment of severe rheumatic disorders. There have been fewer formal trials of chlorambucil, but there is a suggestion that it may be as effective as cyclophosphamide with fewer side-effects.

6.1 Absorption

It is well absorbed with rapid attainment of peak blood levels and a short plasma half-life. There is very little pharmacokinetic data available.

6.2 Side-effects and Toxicity

Side-effects are similar to those of cyclophosphamide, but haemorrhagic cystitis and alopecia do not occur. The principal problems are bone marrow suppression, infections, gastrointestinal disturbances and stomatitis. The same potential problems of oncogenesis, mutagenesis, dysmorphogenicity and infertility exist as with cyclophosphamide.

6.3 Clinical Use

The same indications are appropriate for cyclophosphamide and chlorambucil. It is the last resort in rheumatoid arthritis for patients who fail to respond to drugs like penicillamine. Ancedotal evidence suggests that it may be useful in children with juvenile chronic polyarthritis complicated by amyloidosis and in patients with systemic lupus erythematosus and progressive renal disease. It is for such patients that chlorambucil should be reserved.

6.4 Preparations and Dosage

Chlorambucil is available as 2 and 5mg tablets. Dosage should be kept to a minimum and about 0.1mg/kg a day is appropriate. Most patients with rheumatoid arthritis require between 2.5 and 7.5mg daily. It is reasonable to start with 5mg daily, reducing in the event of neutropenia to a lower dose.

6.5 Cautions

The same cautions as for cyclophosphamide apply to the use of chlorambucil.

7. Methotrexate

Methotrexate is 4-amino-10-methylfolic acid. It is an antimetabolite which acts by binding to the enzyme dihydrofolate reductase and thus inhibiting the conversion of dihydrofolic acid (formed from folic acid) to tetrahydrofolic acid. This interferes with the synthesis of DNA in cells. The drug is therefore active only on cells which are in a DNA-synthesising phase. It has been used to treat psoriasis, psoriatic arthropathy and polymyositis.

7.1 Absorption, Distribution and Elimination

Methotrexate is well absorbed from the gastrointestinal tract after small oral doses ($< 30mg/m^2$) but poorly absorbed after large doses ($> 80mg/m^2$). About a third of an oral dose undergoes metabolism by intestinal bacteria during absorption, thereby reducing bioavailability. It is about 50% bound to plasma proteins. It has a plasma elimination half-life ranging from 6 to 69 hours (mean 27h). Methotrexate is excreted mainly unchanged in urine but to a lesser extent also in bile. It is actively secreted in the renal tubule by the organic acid transport system. Renal clearance is correlated with endogenous creatinine clearance and may provide a guide to dose adjustment according to renal function and age.

7.2 Drug Interactions

Salicylates reduce the clearance rate of methotrexate and may increase the risk of toxicity. Phenylbutazone also enhances the toxicity of methotrexate, presumably by delaying renal elimination (see section 2.3). These potential interactions with aspirin and phenylbutazone are of particular relevance is psoriatic arthropathy.

7.3 Side-effects and Toxicity

Methotrexate may cause gastrointestinal intolerance, particularly diarrhoea, mouth ulceration, leucopenia or thrombocytopenia, infertility, megaloblastic anaemia and skin changes including dermatitis, photosensitivity, alopecia and depigmentation. Hepatic fibrosis has been reported in patients with psoriasis after long-term therapy, although the exact role of methotrexate in this is uncertain. The risk is probably low in patients treated with low doses or for short periods. Liver function tests are not a good guide to its development, detection of which requires liver biopsy.

7.4 Clinical Use

Methotrexate is used for difficult cases of psoriasis and for psoriatic arthropathy. There is an impression that it may be more effective than azathioprine for skin disease but less effective for joint disease. It has also been used in polymyositis for patients resistant to corticosteroids.

7.5 Preparations and Dosage

Methotrexate is available as a 2.5mg tablet. It is probably best given in a single weekly dose of 10 to 25mg before food. It can also be given by intramuscular injection. Dosage must be reduced in patients with impaired renal function.

7.6 Cautions

Regular blood counts are essential in patients receiving methotrexate with close observation for other side-effects.

References and Recommended Reading

Gold

Arthritis and Rheumatism Council. Annals of Rheumatic Diseases 19: 95 (1960).

Gerber, R.C. and Paulus, H.E.: Gold therapy. Clinics in Rheumatic Diseases 1: 307 (1975).

Lorber, A.: Monitoring gold plasma levels in rheumatoid arthritis. Clinical Pharmacokinetics 2: 127 (1977).

Lorber, A.; Atlans, C.J.; Chang, C.C.; Lee, Y.B.; Starrs, J. and Bovy, R.A.: Monitoring serum gold values to improve chrysotherapy in rheumatoid arthritis. Annals of the Rheumatic Diseases 32: 133 (1973).

Research Sub-Committee of The Empire Rheumatism Council. Gold therapy in rheumatoid arthritis. Final report of a multicentre controlled trial. Annals of the Rheumatic Diseases 20: 315 (1961).

Rothermich, N.O.; Philips, V.K.; Bergen, W. and Thomas, M.H.: Chrysotherapy. A prospective study. Arthritis and Rheumatism 19: 1321 (1976).

Sigler, J.W.; Bluhm, G.B.; Duncan, H.; Sharp, J.T.; Ensign, D.C. and McCrum;, W.R.: Gold salts in the treatment of rheumatoid arthritis. Annals of Internal Medicine 80: 21 (1974).

Vorenkamp, E.O. and de Blecourt, J.J.: VIII Rheumatism Conference, Brighton, England.

D-Penicillamine

Day, A.T.; Golding, J.R.; Lee, P.N. and Butterworth, Ann D.: Penicillamine in rheumatoid disease: A long term study. British Medical Journal 1: 180 (1974).

Huskisson, E.C.: Penicillamine and the rheumatologist: a review. Pharmatherapeutica 1: 24 (1976).

Jaffe, I.A.: The treatment of rheumatoid arthritis and necrotizing vasculitis with penicillamine. Arthritis and Rheumatism 13: 436 (1970).

Lyle, W.H. and Kleiman, R.L. (Eds): Penicillamine at 21: Its place in therapeutics now. Proceedings of the Royal Society of Medicine 70: Suppl. 3 (1977).

Multicentre Trial Group: Controlled trial of D-penicillamine in severe rheumatoid arthritis. Lancet 1: 275 (1973).

Azathioprine

Currey, H.L.F.; Harris, J.; Mason, R.M.; Woodland, J.; Beveridge, T.; Roberts, C.J.; Vere, D.W.; Dixon, A. St. J.; Davies, J. and Owen-Smith, B.: Comparison of azathioprine, cyclophosphamide, and gold in treatment of rheumatoid arthritis. British Medical Journal 3: 763 (1974).

Urowitz, M.B.; Gordon, D.A. and Broder, I.: Studies into the occurrence of soluble antigen-antibody complexes in disease. V. Second assessment of correlation between the rheumatoid biologically active factor (RBAF) and the clinical features of rheumatoid arthritis. Arthritis and Rheumatology 16: 225 (1973).

Chloroquine and Hydroxychloroquine

Arden, G.B. and Kolb, H.: Antimalarial therapy and early retinal changes in patients with rheumatoid arthritis. British Medical Journal 1: 270 (1966).

Hart, C.W. and Naunton, R.F.: The ototoxicity of chloroquine phosphate. Archives of Otolaryngology 80: 407 (1964).

Laaksonen, A.L.; Koskiahde, V. and Juka, K.: Dosage of antimalarial drugs for children with juvenile rheumatoid arthritis and systemic lupus erythematosus. A clinical study with determination of serum concentrations of chloroquine and hydroxychloroquine. Scandinavian Journal of Rheumatology 3: 103 (1974).

Popert, A.J.; Meijers, K.A.E.; Sharp, J. and Bier, F.: Chloroquine diphosphate in rheumatoid athritis. Annals of the Rheumatic Diseases 20: 18 (1961).

Cyclophosphamide

Currey, H.L.F.; Harris, J.; Mason, R.M.; Woodland, J.; Beveridge, T.; Roberts, C.J.; Vere, D.W.; Dixon, A. St. J.; Davies, J. and Owen-Smith, B.: Comparison of azathioprine, cyclophosphamide, and gold in treatment of rheumatoid arthritis. British Medical Journal 3: 763 (1974).

Cooperating Clinics Committee of the American Rheumatism Association: A controlled trial of cyclophosphamide in rheumatoid arthritis. New England Journal of Medicine 283: 883 (1970).

Pearson, C.M. and Levy, J.: Immunosuppressive drugs: Mechanism of action, toxicity and clinical effects. Clinics in Rheumatic Diseases 1: 459 (1975).

Chlorambucil

Snaith, M.L.; Holt, J.M.; Oliver, D.O.; Dunnill, M.S.; Halley, W. and Stephenson, A.C.: Treatment of patients with systemic lupus erythematosus including nephritis with chlorambucil. British Medical Journal 2: 197 (1973).

Methotrexate

Metzger, A.L.; Bohan, A.; Goldberg, L.S.; Bluestone, R. and Pearson, C.M.: Polymyositis and dermatomyositis: Combined methotrexate and corticosteroid therapy. Annals of Internal Medicine 81: 182 (1974).

Weinstein, G.D. and Frost, P.: Methotrexate for psoriasis. A new therapeutic schedule. Archives of Dermatology 103: 33 (1971).

Chapter IV

Systemic Corticosteroids and Corticotrophin

The corticosteroids have such a wide range of action in the body that it would be easier to state what actions they don't have than to say what they do to various body processes. They influence carbohydrate, fat, protein and purine metabolism, electrolyte and water balance, and affect all the various systems of the body, particularly the musculoskeletal, renal, endocrinological and cardiovascular systems and tissues. A given dose may have a physiological or pharmacological action, depending on the size of the dose and the physiological or pathological state of the patient at the time.

The following discussion is confined to corticosteroid action relevant to the rheumatic disorders only. Although corticosteroids have a dramatic effect on a variety of disorders where hypersensitivity plays a large part, there is no good evidence that at therapeutic doses they have any real effect on circulating antibodies, either IgG or IgE, in various allergic or autoimmune states; their therapeutic effect being more on prevention or suppression of the inflammation that results from these reactions.

1. Anti-inflammatory Action of the Corticosteroids

All the cardinal clinical features of inflammation — local heat, redness, swelling and tenderness — are prevented or diminished by corticosteroids. This is seen most vividly in their use in inflammatory allergic conditions of the conjunctivum. They inhibit not only the early microscopical features of oedema, capillary dilatation, phagocyte activity, leucocyte migration and fibrin deposition, but also the later features of capillary and fibroblast proliferation, deposition of collagen and finally scarring. This applies whatever may be the cause of the inflammation, mechanical, infective, allergic or immunological; their therapeutic effects being therefore entirely non-specific and palliative, suppressive and temporary.

This anti-inflammatory action may be entirely beneficial but may also be extremely dangerous if active infecting agents are present. The corticosteroids have no antibacterial or antiviral action, although they may appear to help by suppressing inflammation and so exposing the infecting agent (for instance, the tubercle bacillus) to effective antibiotic action, rather, as it has been said, like the beaters on a shoot flattening the brush and putting up the birds for the sportsmen to shoot down. They may also make the patient appear so much better that the true diagnosis of the underlying infection is missed, with fatal results. As Haynes and Larner (1975) grimly commented, corticosteroids misused may permit a patient to walk all the way to the autopsy room. Nevertheless, used correctly, they are the most effective anti-inflammatory agents we have at our disposal. How they act in rheumatic disorders is obscure. The lysosomal stabilisation hypothesis (Weissman and Thomas, 1968) popular previously, does not satisfy all investigators (Haynes and Larner, 1975; Haynes, 1975).

2. Prednisolone

Prednisolone, 11β, 17α, 21-trihydroxypregna-1, 4-diene-3, 20-dione, will be taken as the prototype compound. With continued therapy above 7.5mg daily endogenous pituitary secretion of corticotrophin is depressed, the adrenal cortex undergoing involution with depression of its secretion. At therapeutic dose levels, prednisolone has less sodium retaining action than cortisone and is therefore much less suitable for use in adrenal cortex deficiency states. The action of prednisolone is temporary and a return of symptoms and signs rapidly occurs on stopping or making major reductions in dosage of the drug, unless the treated condition has spontaneously subsided.

2.1 Absorption, Distribution and Elimination

Prednisolone is rapidly absorbed from the gastrointestinal tract and to a smaller and variable extent from other sites, such as synovial spaces, the conjunctival sac and skin. The corticosteroids are reversibly bound to plasma proteins under normal circumstances (Mills et al., 1960). Two protein fractions are involved; one an α-glycoprotein (corticosteroid binding globulin), the other plasma albumin. Corticosteroid binding globulin has a high affinity but low capacity for certain corticosteroids. When the binding capacity of the globulin is exceeded, binding takes place increasingly to albumin, which has low affinity but high capacity for corticosteroids such as cortisol and prednisolone. Thus, at low or normal plasma concentrations, prednisolone is largely bound to the globulin; with increasing levels, the globulin bound corticosteroid changes little, but the fraction of free and albumin bound corticosteroid increases. This has important implications in therapy.

Hypoalbuminaemic states, with their consequent diminution in storage capacity for prednisolone, can with high dose therapy lead to unusually high levels of free unbound drug and enhanced susceptibility to steroid side-effects. With high doses, the percentage of bound prednisolone decreases about 50% when serum albumin falls from 4g/100ml to 2.5g/100ml (Lewis et al., 1971). Prednisolone binding is less complete and less firm than that of cortisol. Corticosteroids can compete with each other for binding sites on the corticosteroid binding globulin.

Prednisolone is rapidly metabolised in the liver, conjugated and excreted in the urine. Although prednisolone disappears from the blood within 100 to 200 minutes, having a half-life of around an hour (Dluhy et al., 1975), its metabolic actions initiated at tissue level persist for many hours. Metabolic degradation is slower with prednisolone than with cortisol.

2.2. Drug Interactions

The rate of metabolism of certain corticosteroids such as dexamethasone, hydrocortisone and methylprednisolone has been reported to be enhanced by phenobarbitone, phenytoin and rifampicin (Brooks et al., 1972; Choi et al., 1971; Edwards et al., 1974; Haque et al., 1972; Stjernholm and Katz, 1975; Werk et al., 1964), probably by inducing hepatic microsomal drug metabolising enzymes. In some reports, the therapeutic efficacy of the steroid (dexamethasone, prednisone, prednisolone, cortisone) has been reduced, as reflected in lack of usual response, increased steroid dose requirements, or steroid toxicity on stopping the enzyme inducing drug (Buffington et al., 1976; Brooks et al., 1972; Boylan et al., 1976; Edwards et al., 1974; Werk et al., 1969).

Concurrent administration of corticosteroids and aspirin decreases plasma salicylate levels due to a more rapid rate of salicylate metabolism so that therapeutic salicylate levels may not be attained (Champion et al., 1977). Klinenberg and Miller (1965) showed that a reduction of corticosteroid dosage in 4 patients resulted in increased plasma salicylate levels in all cases, with symptoms of salicylate intoxication in one. The risk of hyperglycaemia and potassium loss is increased by concurrent therapy with corticosteroids and thiazide and related diuretics. Corticosteroids may make control of diabetes with insulin or oral hypoglycaemic drugs more difficult.

2.3. Toxic Effects

The so-called toxic effects are all too commonly the effects of overdosage. Almost all doses recommended in almost all text books for almost all disorders will in time produce some or all of the features of Cushing's disease. The complications of corticosteroid therapy (table I) have been well reviewed by David et al. (1971). The 3 major types of adverse effects are given by Dujoune and Azarnoff (1975) as:

1) Adrenal insufficiency following withdrawal of therapy, due to continued inhibition of hypothalamic adrenal corticotrophin releasing factor and/or adrenal atrophy from previous corticosteroid therapy.

2) Iatrogenic hyperadrenocorticism, leading to the features of Cushing's disease.

3) Reactivation of the disease process that has been suppressed on stopping or reducing therapy.

Other possible adverse effects of systemic corticosteroids are numerous but those of most importance include:

4) Impaired carbohydrate metabolism. The corticosteroids stimulate gluconeogenesis, primarily through a catabolic (or antianabolic) action on protein. They appear to antagonise the action of insulin at a cellular level and therefore may aggravate or induce diabetes mellitus. The so-called steroid diabetes is usually mild and ketosis is rare.

5) Facilitation of growth and spread of many micro-organisms: viruses, bacteria, fungi, etc.

6) Pseudotumour cerebri. The patient, usually a child, develops papilloedema during treatment which is usually reversed on stopping corticosteroids but sometimes appears with dose reduction, particularly with triamcinolone (Eckler et al., 1966).

7) Psychiatric changes: insomnia, nervousness, mania, depression, even schizophrenia and suicidal attempts. It is possible that such adverse effects are more likely to occur in persons with pre-existing personality disorders, but they may be seen on occasion in apparently normal subjects.

8) Glaucoma and cataract formation.

9) Peptic and intestinal ulceration and perforation.

10) Pancreatitis (rare).

11) Growth retardation in children. Although rheumatoid arthritis may suppress and delay normal growth, natural or therapeutic remission of arthritic disease induced by other therapeutic agents will lead to a return of natural growth, but continued corticosteroid therapy leads to persistent stunting if such therapy cannot be drastically reduced or discontinued.

12) Osteoporosis and spontaneous fractures.

13) Aseptic bone necrosis.

14) Myopathy.

15) Vasculitis and neuropathy. It is the author's and other workers' impression that vasculitis and neuropathy occur more commonly in rheumatoid arthritis in corticosteroid-treated patients, particularly with erratic and irregular dosage (Hart, 1966, 1976; Kemper et al., 1957).

Patients who have received corticosteroid therapy for more than a few weeks at any but minimal dosage (under 7.5mg daily prednisolone or equivalent), must be con-

Table I. Adverse effects of systemic corticosteroids

1. *Endocrine:* Adrenal suppression; hypotension; lack of energy; hyperglycaemia and glycosuria ('steroid diabetes mellitus'); hirsutism; amenorrhoea; growth retardation in children.
2. *Electrolyte disturbances:* Hypokalaemia, sodium and fluid retention; hypertension.
3. *Muscles:* Myopathy.
4. *Bone and Joints:* Infection; aseptic necrosis; osteoporosis.
5. *CNS:* Headaches; mental and mood changes; intracranial hypertension.
6. *Eye:* Posterior subcapsular cataract; glaucoma; papilloedema.
7. *Gastrointestinal:* Gastroduodenal upsets; peptic ulcer exacerbation and perforation; intussesception; perforated diverticula.
8. *Skin and subcutanous tissues:* Atropy; 'steroid purpura'; moon face; acne; redistribution of body fat; increased 'buffalo hump'; increased tendency to infection.

sidered as having in all probability an impaired response to stress. Oyama (1969) noted that such patients given general anaesthesia tended to develop arterial hypotension if not given an adequate corticosteroid supplement prior to and during anaesthesia. To raise the dose in patients on corticosteroid therapy in the face of major stress of any kind is usual practice, i.e. before and during any major surgery or severe intercurrent illness, such as coronary occlusion. Since such adrenocortical suppression may continue for up to 6 months after stopping treatment, many physicians give corticosteroids in the face of any major stress during this period, though it may in fact, in many cases be unnecessary.

Pregnancy in women on corticosteroids does not appear to increase the toxic effects in the mother, but there are different views in regard to risk to the fetus. Warrell and Taylor (1968) compared 34 pregnancies of mothers on corticosteroids with those of an equal number of matched patients not on corticosteroids. 8 stillbirths and 5 cases of placental insufficiency were found in the treated, as opposed to 1 and 3 respectively in the control group. Yackel et al. (1966), on the other hand, in a review of records of 21 deliveries, found no damage to the fetus. Wilson (1973) in a review of drugs as dysmorphogens in man considered corticosteroids to have little or no dysmorphogenic risk.

The evidence alleging an increased incidence of cleft palate when corticosteroids are used in early pregnancy is not convincing. Some 15 years ago, the author sent a questionnaire to all the main rheumatism units in Great Britain asking for details of congenital abnormalities in children born of mothers who had conceived while on corticosteroids and been on corticosteroid therapy during early pregnancy. None were reported, Popert (1976) observing no fetal abnormalities in 13 normal full-term babies of normal birth weight. Corticosteroid therapy should be continued in a pregnant mother for whom it is necessary. Prednisolone is excreted in very small quantities in breast milk and appears to be of no consequence to the nursing infant.

2.4 Clinical Use

The uses of corticosteroids are many, but if we confine this description to the rheumatic disorders they are described in detail under the different disorders. A few points may, however, be made in relation to some of these disorders. Essentially, their practical use is as highly effective anti-inflammatory agents to control the inflammatory features of the various disorders in joints, arteries and other tissues.

2.4.1 Rheumatoid Arthritis

The corticosteroids are only used in this disorder when inflammatory features dominate, and when these inflammatory features have not responded to other non-steroidal agents and to simple physical measures such as rest and splintage. The bad reputation the corticosteroids earned in the 1950s in this disorder was essentially due to dosage being pitched too high. A dramatic response and a very grateful patient (the honeymoon phase) gradually gave way to a rheumatoid patient with iatrogenic Cushing's disease (the chronic unhappy matrimonial phase) and in a few cases to death (divorce).

There is considerable evidence that if dosage exceeds 6 to 7mg daily of prednisolone (or equivalent) in this disease some side-effects will eventually follow. It is far easier to start corticosteroid therapy than to stop it. In other disorders such as asthma or acute systemic lupus erythematosus, a higher dosage may well be better tolerated with fewer side-effects. Some active inflammatory rheumatoids may tolerate the drug well at high dosage initially, but generally speaking daily dosage of 7mg often, and 10mg invariably, will be followed by unwanted features of overdosage within a few weeks or months. A single dose of 5mg at night may improve the night pains, and morning stiffness in rheumatoid arthritis. Although it has been shown that such an evening dose suppresses secretion of corticotrophin more than a morning dose, one has to balance clinical improvement and the patient's opinion against laboratory findings.

Alternate day therapy is advocated by some workers as less likely to produce hypophthalamic-pituitary-adrenal (HPA) axis suppression but patients almost always prefer daily therapy as symptoms tend to recur on the second (off) day. Grant et al. (1965) showed that a single morning dose of corticosteroid produces less suppression of 17-hydroxycorticosteroids than the same total dose given 4 times daily, but again, it is the clinical response that determines the mode of dosage. Myles et al. (1971) found most rheumatoid patients could be managed satisfactorily on a single morning dose of corticosteroids.

Injectable intramuscular prednisolone has been suggested to avoid misuse by the patient, but is is more unpleasant for the patient and gives the physician rather less certain control over the clinical condition than the oral route because of variable absorption from different injection sites (Kettel and Morse, 1975).

2.4.2 Systemic Lupus Erythematosus (SLE)

Corticosteroids are the main weapon in the treatment of this condition, and Dubois (1974) lists the response to therapy of the different clinical features of the disease in his series of 409 cases, comparing results with the series of 62 patients reported by Harvey et al. (1954). Comparison of the results in these 2 large series demonstrates how most of the acute features of the disease are controlled relatively rapidly, given adequate dosage. Dubois (1974) comments, however, that corticosteroids may have negligible effects on severe myocarditis, renal disease and cerebral vasculitis. Although larger amounts of prednisolone produce a more rapid response, dosage tends to be more conservative today than it was some years ago. At high dosage, therapeutic complications increase and intercurrent infections are more common. It is not uncommon to see the fever of infection replacing that of active lupus and as the clinical manifestations are suppressed such infections are always dangerous and sometimes fatal.

According to Yount et al. (1975), the primary mechanism of tissue injury in SLE seems to be the inflammatory response induced by local activation of complement components at sites of tissue deposition. Corticosteroids would appear to do no more than suppress the inflammatory reaction, having no lasting or permanent effect on the underlying pathology (see further chapter XIII).

2.4.3 Other Rheumatic Conditions

The use of corticosteroids in other rheumatic conditions is as described under the different disease states. In rheumatic fever corticosteroids take second place to salicylates. Even given early in large doses, corticosteroids do not appear to prevent or minimise cardiac damage. They effectively reverse the acute exudative phase and are probably more potent in this respect than salicylates, but because of side-effects are usually restricted to severe cases or cases intolerant of, or poorly responding to, salicylates.

2.4.4 Polymyalgia Arteritica

In polymyalgia arteritica, corticosteroids are the drug of choice and probably the only agents that, given in time and at adequate dosage, will prevent the development of blindness (see chapter XII).

2.5 Preparations and Dosage

Prednisolone is available as tablets of 1 and 5mg, the former being used for gradual minimal dose reduction, as in withdrawal in rheumatoid arthritis and polymyalgia arteritica. Enteric coated tablets of 2.5mg are useful in dyspeptic patients. Soluble tablets of prednisolone disodium phosphate (5mg) dissolved in water may be preferred. Dosage will depend entirely on the condition to be treated, the general rule being to use the lowest daily dose which adequately suppresses the disorder. In rheumatoid arthritis, for instance, daily dosage continued over 7mg daily will eventually produce some undesirable side-effects. In each individual case, therapeutic effect and possible toxicity have to be assessed and balanced against each other; the more dangerous the condition (e.g. SLE and giant cell arteritis), the higher the dosage permitted. Cautions and contraindications are also relative to the individual case.

2.6 Cautions

Intercurrent infections; diabetes mellitus; mental instability. Congestive heart failure. Corticosteroids should not be suddenly withdrawn as symptoms of the suppressed disease may flare up in acute form. Corticosteroids should be avoided in active pulmonary tuberculosis (relative); manic depressive psychoses; active peptic ulceration; and severe osteoporosis in immobilised patients.

2.7 Alternative Corticosteroids

Prednisone and prednisolone are interchangeable in therapeutics and in the body. Prednisone is converted to the active form prednisolone by the liver. This biotransformation may be decreased in the presence of severe disease of the liver (Powell and Axelsen, 1972), but the two agents for practical purposes may be considered identical. Prednisone is prescribable in tablets of 5 and 1mg.

Methylprednisolone is available as 2, 4 and 16mg tablets. The larger strength tablets are intended for alternate day therapy (see above).

Triamcinolone is available as tablets of 1, 2 and 4mg. It has virtually no sodium retaining effect and during the first few days of therapy may cause sodium loss in the urine and act as a mild diuretic. Bizarre symptoms, such as nausea, weight loss and dizziness may occur occasionally.

Dexamethasone is available as tablets of 0.5, 0.75 and 2mg.

Betamethasone is available as 0.5mg tablets and as soluble betamethasone sodium phosphate 0.5mg tablets.

Paramethasone is available as 2mg tablets.

Cortisone and *hydrocortisone* are more suited for adrenal replacement therapy and less suitable for antirheumatic (anti-inflammatory) treatment because of their greater sodium retaining effect.

There is usually little or no advantage in substituting any of the above for oral systemic therapy with prednisone or prednisolone. An equivalent anti-inflammatory effect is obtained with approximately 25mg cortisone, 20mg hydrocortisone (cortisol), 4mg prednisone or prednisolone, 4mg triamcinolone or methylprednisolone, 2mg paramethasone and 0.75mg dexamethasone or betamethasone. Triamcinolone, paramethasone, dexamethasone and betamethasone have virtually no sodium retaining potency at usual dose levels.

3. Corticotrophin (ACTH)

Human corticotrophin is a peptide of 39 amino-acid residues. It stimulates the human adrenal cortex to secrete cortisol, corticosterone, aldosterone and a number of weak androgenic substances. Prolonged administration therefore produces adrenocortical hyperplasia and increased synthesis and output of cortisol. Corticotrophin is derived from the pituitaries of animals used for human food. It is ineffective given orally, as it is destroyed by the proteolytic enzymes of the gastrointestinal tract.

ACTH activity resides largely in the first 24 amino-acids of the peptide chain which are identical in pig, sheep, cow and human. It is stored in protein bound and free forms in the pituitary. ACTH is readily absorbed after intramuscular injection and after intravenous administration. It rapidly disappears from the circulation; in man the plasma half-life being around 15 minutes. It is inactivated in the tissues, no biological activity being present in the urine.

3.1 Toxic Effects

These are, apart from hypersensitivity reactions such as fever and anaphylaxis, as under prednisolone — with a greater incidence of hypertension, heart strain, acne, sodium loading and hypokalaemic alkalosis. When allergic reactions occur, therapeutic effects diminish, sometimes dramatically. Antibodies may develop to corticotrophin on prolonged therapy (Glass and Daly, 1971).

3.2 Clinical Use

The indications for use of ACTH are as under prednisolone. Following courses of intramuscular injections of corticotrophin, hypothalamic and pituitary activity is suppressed but adrenal responsiveness is retained. Booster doses of corticotrophin, used in the past in patients on prolonged corticosteroid oral therapy in an attempt to prevent suppression of the adrenal cortex, failed to do so; Carter and James (1970) finding increased suppression of the HPA axis rather than the reverse. A course of 1 to 3 weeks of intramusuclar corticotrophin may be given to patients in hospital in acute relapse of any acute inflammatory arthropathy, in the hope that the condition will settle, rather than starting corticosteroids by mouth, with all the attendant difficulties later of withdrawal or dose control.

3.3 Preparations and Dosage

Corticotrophin is available in a number of forms: (1) hydrolysed gelatin, 20, 40 and 80 international units per ml for intramuscular or subcutaneous use; (2) absorbed on zinc hydroxide, 40 international units per ml; and (3) complexed with and dissolved in carboxylethylcellulose, 20 and 40 international units per ml.

These repository forms are given once daily. Dosage depends on the condition to be treated, averaging 10 to 40 international units; higher dosage is permissible in severe and intractable conditions. For intravenous use, sterile solutions of corticotrophin are available where more intense adrenocortical stimulation is required, maximum stimulation being obtained in adults with 25 units infused over a period of 8 hours.

3.4 Cautions and Contraindications

These are as with prednisolone. Because of its mineralocorticoid action it should not be used in patients with hypertension and/or left heart strain. Acne will be aggravated. Although gastrointestinal complications may be less than with oral corticosteroids they do occur. Allergic reactions are sometimes severe and, rarely, may be fatal.

4. Tetracosactrin

Tetracosactrin is a synthetic analogue of corticotrophin; it contains the first 24 of the 39 amino-acids and has the complete therapeutic activity of corticotrophin. Tetracosactrin has the therapeutic and the undesirable effects described under corticotrophin. Although allergic reactions may be less common, local tissue reactions may occur and Glass et al. (1971) noted the development of antibodies in 12 of 38 patients treated over several months. It is available as tetracosacrtin zinc complex (long-acting form) 1mg per ml ampoule and 2mg per 2ml multi-dose vial and may be given by intramuscular injection daily or every few days. Small doses such as 0.1 to 0.15mg daily are more effective in reducing arthritic symptoms than larger injections such as 0.25 to 0.50mg given every 3 to 4 days. Whatever the frequency of injections, patients receiving doses greater than 1mg tetracosacrtin weekly are likely to develop signs of overdosage, and therapy in the chronic arthritic diseases should, if given over periods of several weeks or months, not exceed 1mg weekly, whether given daily or less frequently.

Tetracosactrin acetate 0.25mg per ml in buffered aqueous solution is also available for intravenous or intramuscular use to test adrenocortical function or to treat anaphylactic shock or drug sensitivity reactions.

As a rough equivalent, 1mg of tetracosactrin given intramuscularly has the clinical effect of 100 to 150 international units of corticotrophin intramuscularly.

References and Recommended Reading

Corticosteroids

Boylan, J.J.; Owen, D.S. and Chin, J.B.: Phenytoin interference with dexamethasone. Journal of the American Medical Association 235: 803 (1976).

Brooks, S.M.; Werk, E.E.; Ackerman, S.J.; Sullivan, Irene and Thrasher, Katherine: Adverse effects of phenobarbital on corticosteroid metabolism in asthmatics. New England Journal of Medicine 286: 1125 (1972).

Buffington, G.A.; Dominguez, H.H.; Piering, W.F.; Hebert, L.A.; Kauffman, H.M. and Lemann, J.: Interaction of rifampicin and glucocorticoids. Journal of the American Medical Association 236: 1958 (1976).

Choi, Y.; Thrasher, K. and Werk, E.E.: Effect of diphenylhydantoin on cortisol kinetics in humans. Journal of Pharmacology and Experimental Therapeutics 176: 27 (1971).

David, D.S.; Grieco, M.H. and Cushman, P.: Adrenal glucocorticoids after twenty years: A review of their clinically relevant consequences. Journal of Chronic Diseases 22: 637 (1971).

Dluhy, R.G.; Newmark, S.R.; Lauler, D.P. and Thron, G.W.: in Azarnoff (Ed) Steroid Therapy, p.8 (Saunders, Philadelphia 1975).

Dujovne, C.A. and Azarnoff, D.L.: in Azarnoff (Ed) Steroid Therapy, p.27 (Saunders, Philadelphia 1975).

Dubois, E.L.: Lupus Erythematosus, 2nd ed, p.163 (University of Southern California Press, Los Angeles 1974).

Eckler, E.; Schonberg, D. and Bierich, J.R.: Monatsschrift fur Kinderheilkunde 114: 271 (1966).

Edwards, O.M.; Courtenay-Evans, R.J.; Galley, J.M.; Hunter, J. and Tait, A.D.: Changes in cortisol metabolism following rifampicin therapy. Lancet 2: 549 (1974).

Graham, G.G.; Champion, G.D.; Day, R.O. and Paull, P.D.: Patterns of plasma concentrations and urinary excretion of salicylate in rheumatoid arthritis. Clinical Pharmacology and Therapeutics 22: 410 (1977).

Grant, S.D.; Forsham, P.H. and Diraimondo, V.C.: Suppression of 17-hydroxycorticosteroids in plasma and urine by single and divided doses of triamcinolone. New England Journal of Medicine 273: 1115 (1965).

Haque, N.; Thrasher, K.; Werk, E.E.; Knowles, H.C. and Sholiton, L.J.: Studies on dexamethasone metabolism in man: effect of diphenylhydantoin. Journal of Clinical Endocrinology and Metabolism 34: 44 (1972).

Hart, F.D.: Complicated rheumatoid disease. British Medical Journal 2: 131 (1966).

Hart, F.D.: in Organic Manifestations and Complications in Rheumatoid Arthritis, p.314 (Schattauer Verlag, Stuttgart 1976).

Harvey, A.M.; Shulman, L.E.; Tumulty, P.A.; Conley, C.L. and Schoenrich, E.H.: Systemic lupus erythematosus: Review of the literature and clinical analysis of 138 cases. Medicine (Baltimore) 33: 291 (1954).

Haynes, R.C. and Larner, J.: in Goodman and Gilman (Eds) The Pharmacological Basis of Therapeutics, 5th ed, p.1488 (Macmillan, New York 1975).

Haynes, R.C.: in Azarnoff (Ed) Steroid Therapy, p.19 (Saunders, Philadelphia 1975).

Kemper, J.W.; Baggenstoss, A.H. and Slocumb, C.H.: The relationship of therapy with cortisone to the incidence of vascular lesions in rheumatoid arthritis. Annals of Internal Medicine 46: 831 (1957).

Kettel, L.J. and Morse, J.O.: in Azarnoff (Ed) Steroid Therapy, p.293 (Saunders, Philadelphia 1975).

Klinenberg, J.R. and Miller, R.: Effect of corticosteroids on blood salicylate concentrations. Journal of the American Medical Association 194: 601 (1965).

Lewis, G.P.; Jusko, W.J.; Burke, C.W. and Graves, Linda: Prednisone side effects and serum protein levels. Lancet 2: 778 (1971).

Mills, I.H.; Schedl, H.P.; Chen, P.S. and Bartter, F.C.: The effect of estrogen administration on the metabolism and protein binding of hydrocortisone. Journal of Clinical Endocrinology and Metabolism 20: 515 (1960).

Myles, A.B.; Bacon, P.A. and Daly, J.R.: Single daily dose corticosteroid treatment. Effect on adrenal function and therapeutic efficacy in various diseases. Annals of the Rheumatic Diseases 30: 149 (1971).

Oyama, T.: Hazards of steroids in association with anaesthesia. Canadian Anaesthetics Society Journal 16: 361 (1969).

Popert, A.J.: Personal communication (1976).

Powell, L.W. and Axelsen, Elizabeth: Corticosteroids in liver disease: Studies on the biological conversion of prednisone to prednisolone and plasma protein binding. Gut 13: 690 (1972).

Stjernholm, M.R. and Katz, F.H.: Effects of diphenylhydantoin, phenobarbital, and diazepam on the metabolism of methylprednisolone and its sodium succinate. Journal of Clinical Endocrinology and Metabolism 41: 887 (1975).

Warrell, D.W. and Taylor, R.: Outcome for the foetus of mothers receiving prednisolone during pregnancy. Lancet 1: 117 (1968).

Weissman, G. and Thomas, R.: Recent Progress in Hormone Research 20: 215 (1968).

Werk, E.E.; Choi, Y.; Sholiton, L.; Olinger, C. and Haque, N.: Interference in the effect of dexamethasone by diphenylhydantoin. New England Journal of Medicine 281: 32 (1969).

Werk, E.E.; MacGee, J. and Sholitan, L.J.: Effect of diphenylhydantoin on cortisol metabolism in man. Journal of Clinical Investigation 43: 1824 (1964).

Wilson, J.G.: Present status of teratogens in man. Teratology 7: 3 (1973).

Yackel, D.S.; Kempers, R.D. and McConahey, W.M.: Adrenocorticosteroid therapy in pregnancy. American Journal of Obstetrics and Gynaecology 96: 985 (1966).

Yount, W.J.; Utsinger, P.D.; Hadler, N.M. and Gammon, W.R.: in Azarnoff (Ed) Steroid Therapy, p.271 (Saunders, Philadelphia 1975).

Corticotrophin

Carter, M.E. and James, V.H.T.: An attempt at combining corticotrophin with long-term corticosteroid therapy. Annals of the Rheumatic Diseases 29: 409 (1970).

Glass, D. and Daly, J.R.: Development of antibodies during long-term therapy with corticotrophin in rheumatoid arthritis. I. Procine ACTH. Annals of the Rheumatic Diseases 30: 589 (1971).

Glass, D.; Nuki, G. and Daly, J.R.: Development of antibodies during long-term therapy with corticotrophin in rheumatoid arthritis. II. Zinc tetracosactrin (depot synacthen). Annals of the Rheumatic Diseases 30: 593 (1971).

Chapter V

Intra-Articular and Soft Tissue Injections

1. Corticosteroids

Corticosteroids are also used to achieve a local anti-inflammatory effect. By giving them intra-articularly, or directly into soft tissues, it is possible to avoid their undesirable systemic effects (see chapt. IV; sect. 2.3). Local injection of a corticosteroid is the treatment of choice in certain soft tissue conditions such as tennis elbow and injection into a joint is a useful adjunct to other forms of therapy for various types of inflammatory arthritis.

1.1 Side-effects

Infection occurs after about 1 in 10,000 intra-articular injections. It demands prompt recognition and treatment with antibiotics and regular needle aspiration to achieve drainage. Destructive changes in the joint surface may follow repeated injections. Crystalline preparations may produce an acute crystal synovitis and the joint is often 'sore' for 24 hours after the procedure. Rest will usually relieve it. Injection of tennis elbows is often exquisitely painful and the pain may last for 1 or 2 days afterwards. It is wise to warn the patient of this and to supply some simple analgesics to be taken if required.

1.2. Clinical Use

The indications for intra-articular and local injection of corticosteroids are summarised in table I.

Table I. Indications for intra-articular and local corticosteroids

1. *Intra-articular*
   a) Relief of pain resulting from inflammatory arthritis localised to one or a few joints.
   b) To aid the mobilisation of a stiff joint.
   c) To aid the correction of deformity.

2. *Local*
   a) The enthesopathies — e.g. tennis elbow.
   b) Compression neuropathies — e.g. carpal tunnel syndrome.
   c) Tenosynovitis.
   d) Epidural injection of steroid has been shown to be a useful treatment in acute lumbar disc prolapse with root compression.

1.2.1 Intra-articular Injection

The most common reason for injecting corticosteroids into a joint is to achieve relief of pain. This treatment is particularly appropriate in a patient who has one outstanding problem joint or who has achieved a remission in most joints, but with one or two remaining active and painful. Rheumatoid arthritis is the most common disease for which this treatment is used, but it may be used in any condition in which the pain is believed to result from inflammation. These include psoriatic arthropathy, enteropathic synovitis, ankylosing spondylitis with peripheral arthritis, Reiter's disease and pyrophosphate arthropathy. Studies in osteoarthrosis have so far failed to show any benefit for intra-articular corticosteroids, although this may be useful in the acute inflammatory episodes which punctuate the course of the disease.

Corticosteroid injection is unlikely to be useful when symptoms are due to mechanical derangement. Thus, patients who are likely to benefit are those with warm swollen joints, with effusions and stiffness in the morning and after periods of inactivity. Those who are unlikely to benefit are those with pain related to movement or exercise, crepitus, instability and severe X-ray changes. It is clearly impossible to inject more than a few joints so that patients with many active joints are better treated in other ways.

A steroid injection is a useful aid to the mobilisation of a stiff joint, again when the stiffness is related to inflammation, rather than to irreversible anatomical changes. This is particularly valuable for the shoulder joint, either in inflammatory arthropathies such as rheumatoid arthritis, or in soft tissue conditions like the 'frozen' painful shoulder. In this situation the joint is injected and after 24 hours rest, a programme of physiotherapy is started.

The third reason for injecting joints is to assist in correcting deformities. A patient with rheumatoid arthritis and a recent flexion deformity of the knee, will often be able to straighten the knee after a steroid injection. Relief of inflammation will also make the task of correcting the deformity easier.

1.2.2 Local Injection

Local corticosteroid injection is the treatment of choice for enthesopathies; i.e. conditions like tennis elbow in which the inflammatory process is localised to the junction of tendon or ligament and bone. Similarly, an injection of corticosteroid is the most satisfactory first line treatment for compression neuropathies such as carpal tunnel syndrome. In this condition, the steroid is injected directly into the carpal tunnel and relieves symptoms in a proportion of cases. In tenosynovitis, the injection is made into the inflamed tendon sheath. An example is de Quervain's tenosynovitis in the thumb. In rheumatoid tenosynovitis, local steroid injection is often useful to relieve pain, to stop 'triggering' and to correct deformities resulting from tendon contractures.

1.2.3 Outcome: Repeat Injections

One injection of prednisolone into a tennis elbow or carpal tunnel is usually sufficient. Relief of symptoms can be expected within 24 hours. Recurrences are not uncommon and in conditions like tennis elbow the injection can be repeated. Recurrent carpal tunnel syndrome is probably best treated by surgical decompression.

Intra-articular injection also produces its maximum effect within a few days of the procedure. The benefit is very variable, some patients achieving dramatic benefit, others having no improvement. In successful cases, the benefits may last for months but often it may be for only a few days. The first injection is usually the most successful. If 1 injection fails the second is unlikely to help and the third almost certainly will not, but this is not always true. The benefits of second and subsequent injections are usually progressively briefer than the benefits of the first. It is therefore unjustifiable to give a 'course' of steroid injections. It may be worth repeating the injection after a week or two if the benefit is slight or incomplete.

1.3 Preparations, Dosage and Technique

Prednisolone is the most common preparation used for intra-articular injection, although equivalent doses of hydrocortisone and other compounds are equally satisfactory. Some corticosteroid preparations are crystalline and will induce an acute crystal synovitis if injected into a joint. It is therefore essential to use a preparation which is specifically recommended for intra-articular or local use. Long-acting preparations such as methylprednisolone acetate and triamcinolone hexacetonide may prolong the effect of intra-articular injection and are particularly useful in chronic diseases like rheumatoid arthritis.

The dose of prednisolone used for intra-articular and local injections depends upon the size of the inflamed area into which the injection is made and varies between 10 and 40mg. Most preparations of corticosteroid for intra-articular injections contain about 20mg per ml of prednisolone or the equivalent. 0.5ml is sufficient for injection into the small joints of the hands or feet and for soft tissue injections in de

Quervain's tenosynovitis or tennis elbow. 1ml is sufficient for medium sized joints such as the wrist or for injection into the carpal tunnel. 2ml are required for larger joints such as the knee.

A strict aseptic technique must be used for intra-articular injection. Infection resulting from this procedure is a major disaster to be avoided at all costs. It is unwise to give repeated injections into the same joint and three in the patient's lifetime is usually regarded as the limit in a disease like rheumatoid arthritis.

Warnings to patient: Two important warnings must be given to the patient after intra-articular steroid injections, especially when the procedure is carried out on an outpatient. Firstly, the patient must be advised to return at once if the joint gets worse, because of the possibility of infection. Secondly, the patient should rest more or less completely for 24 hours after injection and thereafter should be advised not to increase his activities greatly, even if the injection is dramatically effective. This particularly applies to weight bearing joints, in which destructive changes may follow repeated intra-articular injections, especially when these are highly successful and when there is a big improvement in the patient's mobility.

For soft tissue injections like tennis elbow, the needle is inserted into the area of maximum tenderness. Techniques of intra-articular injection are described elsewhere (Huskisson and Hart, 1975; Cawley, 1974; Ehrlich, 1973). In the presence of a large effusion in rheumatoid arthritis, it is advisable to aspirate as much fluid as possible before injecting the corticosteroid. In general, best results are seen where aspiration of generous amounts precedes corticosteroid injection.

1.4 Cautions

The most important contraindication to intra-articular corticosteroid injection is the presence of infection in the joint. A patient with rheumatoid arthritis who develops a septic arthritis may present with a single joint which is rather more painful than the rest and it is tempting to inject it. If there is any suspicion of infection the joint must first be aspirated and the results of culture awaited before a corticosteroid injection is given. It is unwise to inject corticosteroid preparations in and around major tendons such as the achilles tendon, especially in athletes, since this seems to predispose to tendon repture. Patients must be instructed carefully after intra-articular corticosteroid injection (section 1.3).

2. Radioactive Colloids

Radioactive colloids are used in joints with the aim of achieving a synovectomy; a dose of localised radiation is applied to the synovium which leads to shrinkage, fibrosis and, as a result, diminished production of synovial fluid. This must be achieved without irradiating other structures such as bone marrow and soft tissues and with the minimum of spread to local lymphatics and other parts of the body. The choice of isotope is determined by these requirements. β-emitters are preferred and they should produce a limited penetration of the surrounding tissues after injection.

Although a number of isotopes have been used in different joints, the most commonly used now is radioactive yttrium (^{90}Y) in the knee joint and this will be considered first.

2.1 Yttrium in the Knee

Yttrium (^{90}Y) seems to be the most suitable isotope for injection into the knee and this is the joint for which radioactive colloids seem to be most used. Although there has been a large amount of uncontrolled study on the value of this treatment, there have been very few controlled trials. One of the latter (Yates et al., 1977) failed to show any benefit from the treatment; another (Bridgman et al., 1973) showed a significant difference in favour of ^{90}Y in terms of joint swelling and movement, but not in other measurements such as pain. The largest numbers of patients have been studied in uncontrolled trials in which the results have been expressed as good, fair etc. These studies suggest that about 60 % of patients obtain a good result, 20 % some improvement, and 20 % no benefit at all. This is, of course, a notoriously unreliable method of assessment and there is a need for more controlled studies before this treatment can be regarded as anything more than an experimental approach. In a recent review of 350 joints, principally knees, treated since December 1970, Gumpel (1977) noted after a minimum period of 3 years had elapsed, that full resolution of synovitis was noted in 40 % of knees and marked improvement in 25 %

2.1.1 Side-effects

Some problems may arise following injection of ^{90}Y, the most common being local pain which occurs in about one third of cases. Other complications occur in about 4 % of cases and include fever and malaise, a local skin eruption, needle track burns, scarring, pigmentation and occasionally radionecrosis. Lymphatic spread occurs in some cases and chromosomal damage has been demonstrated in patients who have received radioactive colloids. The significance of this will not be known until patients receiving this treatment have been followed-up for many years to exclude an excess of malignancy. To date there is no evidence for this.

2.1.2 Clinical Use

Experience suggests that ^{90}Y is particularly useful in cases of persistently active inflammatory rheumatoid arthritis and especially in cases with large and troublesome effusions. It seems that better results have been obtained in seropositive rheumatoid than in seronegative cases, and better results in rheumatoid arthritis than in psoriatic arthropathy and the other seronegative spondylarthropathies. However, some authors have reported good results in a reasonable proportion of cases of diseases other than rheumatoid arthritis, even in osteoarthrosis, a condition in which inflammation is not particularly prominent. Better results are obtained in early cases with active inflammation than in late cases where the symptoms are mainly of mechanical origin. Thus, the presence of soft tissue swelling, effusion and stiffness in the morning and after sitting are good signs, while pain on exercise, crepitus and instability suggest mechanical problems which are likely to persist even if inflammation is controlled.

The patient's progress should be assessed after about 6 months — this seems to be the time at which maximum improvement is achieved. If the result is not satisfactory, the injection may be repeated, but in most patients it will be necessary to consider some alternative therapy.

2.1.3 Dose and Technique

3m Ci of ^{90}Y seems to be the ideal dosage. Larger doses (6m Ci) have been shown to be no more effective and increase in dosage beyond this level may lead to greater hazards. The technique of injection is of the greatest importance. The usual precautions must be taken in dealing with radioactive material, such as disposal of syringes and swabs in the appropriate place. Full aseptic precautions must also be taken for the injection. Following injection, the joint should be immobilised in a splint for 3 days to reduce the lymphatic spread of isotope. Some authors recommend combining ^{90}Y with local anaesthetic, to reduce the pain of the injection, and with corticosteroid. One study (Goode and Howey, 1973) showed that giving corticosteroid intra-articularly 2 days before injection of ^{90}Y reduced the leakage of isotope from the knee and this may be preferable. ^{90}Y does not seem to find its way into the patient's urine so that it is not necessary to take any precautions with this.

2.1.4 Cautions

Because of the dangers of radioactivity, ^{90}Y should not be used in patients under 45 years of age and certainly never in pregnancy, or where the possibility of future pregnancy exists.

2.2 Other Isotopes — Other Joints

The results of injection of isotopes into other joints seem to be less good than those of injection of ^{90}Y into the knee. There are also fewer indications for this type of treatment in other joints. Radioactive erbium (^{169}Er) had been used in the small joints of the hand in doses of 0.25 to 0.5m Ci. Yttrium must not be used for the finger joints since it may cause radionecrosis. Radioactive gold (^{198}Au) has been used but rhenium (^{186}Re) may be preferable. It is used in a dose of 1m Ci for the wrist, 2m Ci for elbows and shoulders, and 3m Ci for the hips. The same precautions must be taken as for the injection of ^{90}Y into the knee.

References and Recommended Reading

Corticosteroids

Cawley, M.I.D.: Arthrocentesis: techniques and indications. British Journal of Hospital Medicine 11: 744 (1974).

Ehrlich, G.E.: Total Management of the Arthritic Patient (Lippincott, Philadelphia 1973).

Huskisson, E.C. and Hart, F.D.: Joint disease. All ther Arthropathies, 2nd ed (John Wright, Bristol 1975).

Radioactive Colloids

Bridgman, J.F.; Bruckner, F.; Eisen, V.; Tucker, A. and Bleehen, N.M.: Irradiation of the synovium in the treatment of rheumatoid arthritis. Quarterly Journal of Medicine 4: 357 (1973).

Goode, J.D. and Howey, S.: Effect of premedication with intra-articular hydrocortisone on the retention of ^{198}Au in the knee joint in rheumatoid arthritis. Use of ^{99m}Tc in assessment. Annals of Rheumatic Diseases 32 (Suppl.): 43 (1973).

Gumpel, J.M.: Review of published and personal results: Criteria for selection of patients. Annals of Rheumatic Diseases 32 (Suppl): 29 (1973).

Gumpel, J.M.: Irradiation of knee with yttrium 90. Results 3 years after treatment. Annals of Rheumatic Diseases 36: 285 (1977).

Ingrand, J.: Characteristics of radio-isotopes for intra-articular therapy. Annals of Rheumatic Diseases 32 (Suppl): 3 (1973).

Yates, D.B.; Scott, J.T. and Ramsey, N.: Double-blind trial of yttrium 90 for chronic inflammatory synovium of the knee. Annals of Rheumatic Diseases 36: 481 (1977).

Chapter VI

Analgesic Drugs

This chapter discusses those agents which relieve pain by a central action on the CNS but have no peripheral anti-inflammatory or so-called 'antirheumatic' action. Some have antipyretic action (paracetamol or acetaminophen), some not (dextropropoxyphene). Aspirin has both an anti-inflammatory and peripheral and central analgesic action and is discussed in chapter II (section 1). At low dose levels, 2g or less daily, the action of aspirin would seem to be largely analgesic.

The place of these analgesics in rheumatology is purely to relieve pain of the rheumatic sufferer and so make life more pleasant and simple essential muscular and joint movements more easy to do. Analgesics are usually given, therefore, in addition to the basic programme of physical measures, rest, exercise and anti-inflammatory and antirheumatic drugs to cover certain 'pain spots' or exertions in the day, when they may be taken to ease the pain or to anticipate it. As a group they are better tolerated, particularly by the gastrointestinal tract, than the non-steroidal anti-inflammatory agents. Although modest in their effects they do help many patients, sometimes, though rarely, considerably. The best analgesic for a sufferer with any chronic painful disorder is an occupied mind. Any time consuming occupation that is meaningful, interesting or rewarding to the patient, however silly it may seem to others, leads to diminished need for 'pain-killers'.

1. Paracetamol

Paracetamol (acetaminophen) is p-acetamidophenol. It has analgesic and antipyretic properties but little or no anti-inflammatory action. It is the major active metabolite of phenacetin and acetanilide, now largely discarded because of their toxic side-effects.

Paracetamol is rapidly and almost completely absorbed from the gastrointestinal tract after oral administration, plasma concentrations reaching a maximum in 30 to 60 minutes. The plasma half-life is 1 to 3 hours. Paracetamol is distributed throughout most body fluids relatively evenly, binding to plasma proteins being very variable. Only about 3% is excreted unchanged in the urine, some 80% being excreted by the kidney after conjugation in the liver, mostly with glucuronic acid. Hydroxylated metabolites are responsible for methaemoglobin formation and liver toxicity. With impaired renal function, only small amounts of unchanged paracetamol are found in the plasma but a larger amount of the conjugated form.

1.1 Drug Interactions

Induction of hepatic microsomal drug metabolising enzymes and potentiation of oral anticoagulants at the usual dosage is negligible, although heavy continuous dosage may affect both processes.

1.2 Side-effects

Paracetamol is usually well tolerated by the gastrointestinal tract and other systems. Overdosage, however, may produce fatal hepatic necrosis (see section 1.5). Thrombocytopenia has been reported; skin rashes and allergic reactions are rare.

1.3 Clinical Use

In the rheumatic disorders paracetamol is used essentially to relieve pain. It is taken as required, usually in addition to regular administration of non-steroidal anti-inflammatory agents. Fever may also be reduced in febrile rheumatic disorders.

1.4 Preparations and Dosage

Tablets contain 500mg, and the usual dose is 1g taken as required up to 3 to 4g daily. Many compound tablets are available.

1.5 Cautions

Paracetamol must not be used in patients with liver disease. Over 7g daily may cause liver damage and larger regular dosage irreversible hepatic necrosis. In suicidal overdosage, death from hepatic necrosis may be delayed several hours, the patient having apparently recovered from the suicidal gesture.

2. Pentazocine

Pentazocine is a benzomorphan derivative. It has an analgesic but no anti-inflammatory action, its main action being on the central nervous system and smooth muscle.

Pentazocine is well absorbed from the gastrointestinal tract and from subcutaneous and intramuscular injection sites, peak plasma levels occurring 1 to 3 hours after oral administration and 15 to 60 minutes after intramuscular administration. The plasma half-life is about 2 hours after intramuscular administration. Duration of action after oral administration is usually 2 to 6 hours. Most of the drug is metabolised in the liver; the metabolites being excreted in the urine along with a small and variable amount of unchanged pentazocine. About 60% of the total dose is excreted within 24 hours.

2.1 Side-effects

Side-effects which occasionally occur include nausea, sedation, sweating, dizziness and rarely hallucinations. High dosage may produce respiratory depression (reversible by naloxone but not nalorphine), tachycardia and hypertension. In some patients, with repeated and frequent use, the analgesic action diminishes, but addiction is rare and it is not on the Misuse of Drugs list in Great Britain (and equivalent list in the USA), whether given by mouth or injection.

2.2 Clinical Use

Pentazocine is a mild analgesic when given orally but is more potent when given by subcutaneous or intramuscular injection.

2.3 Preparations and Dosage

Pentazocine is available as tablets of 25mg and capsules of 50mg, also as ampoules of 30 and 60mg (1 and 2ml) for subcutaneous or intramuscular injection. Oral adult dosage is 25 to 100mg 3 to 4 hourly after meals, as required. Suppositories containing 50mg are also available.

2.4 Cautions

There is considerable individual variation in extent of hepatic metabolism and therapeutic effect. Addiction, though rare, may occur in certain individuals, often previously addicted to other drugs; this occurs largely with the use of parenteral preparations. Pentazocine should be used with great care in pregnancy, in patients with impaired renal, hepatic or respiratory function, or with monoamine oxidase inhibitors or alcohol, or after large doses of narcotic analgesics.

Pentazocine is contraindicated in narcotic addicts; respiratory depression; raised intracranial pressure, head injury or pathological conditions of the brain, or after coronary occlusion where it may cause a rise in pulmonary artery pressure.

3. Dextropropoxyphene

Dextropropoxyphene is (+)-a-4-dimethylamino-3-methyl-1-1,2-diphenyl-but-2yl propionate. It has a central analgesic but no antipyretic or anti-inflammatory action. It is readily absorbed from the gastrointestinal tract; plasma levels are apparent at 1 hour, maximal at about 2 hours, thereafter slowly declining over a further 3 to 4 hours, but there is considerable individual variability. It has a plasma half-life of 12 hours. The major route of metabolism in man is N-demethylation to yield norpropoxyphene, which is excreted in the urine.

3.1 Side-effects

Toxicity is negligible at therapeutic dosage. However, at excessive dosage, central nervous system, cardiac and respiratory depression may occur and sometimes convulsions. Combinations with paracetamol cause major treatment problems on overdosage (Whittington, 1977; Editorial, 1977). Continued administration of 800mg or more daily may cause toxic psychoses or convulsions.

3.2 Clinical Use

Dextropropoxyphene is used solely in the rheumatic diseases for its analgesic effect, taken as required; up to 260mg of the hydrochloride or 400mg of the napsylate daily in divided dosage.

3.3 Preparations

Capsules of dextropropoxyphene napsylate 100mg (equivalent to 65mg of the hydrochloride). There are also many combinations with aspirin, paracetamol etc. available, and a sustained release capsule containing 150mg dextropropoxyphene for use 8 to 12-hourly as required.

3.4 Cautions

Dextropropoxyphene only rarely causes tolerance, euphoria or drug dependence. Nevertheless, it is a narcotic analgesic and its depressant effect may be additive if given with other central nervous depressants, impairing mental and/or physical abilities required for the performance of tasks such as driving a car or operating machinery.

4. Codeine

Codeine has a mild analgesic action and causes constipation. It has a plasma half-life of 2 hours and a duration of action of 4 to 6 hours. Once absorbed, codeine is metabolised by the liver and mainly excreted in inactive forms in the urine. About 10% of a given dose is demethylated to form morphine.

4.1 Side-effects

Codeine constipates at ordinary dose levels and at high levels causes respiratory depression.

4.2 Clinical Use

Codeine is used in the rheumatic disorders as a mild analgesic (usually in combination with other more effective analgesics such as aspirin) and to control diarrhoea. It is useful in those arthropathies associated with diarrhoea (e.g. colitic arthropathies).

4.3 Preparations and Dosage

Codeine is available as the phosphate in tablets. The dosage ranges from 10 to 60mg daily in divided doses. The dose in compound analgesic tablets is usually 5 to 10mg per tablet.

4.4 Cautions

Use with caution in patients with constipation.

5. Dihydrocodeine

Dihydrocodeine tartrate is an analgesic of greater potency than codeine but less than morphine. Sedation is less than with morphine. It is readily absorbed from the gastrointestinal tract and after intramuscular injection, excretion being mostly via the kidneys within 24 hours of administration. Duration of therapeutic action is about 4 to 6 hours.

5.1 Side-effects

Taken by mouth there is little risk of addiction: by intramuscular injection dihydrocodeine is potentially addictive and is controlled under the Misuse of Drugs Act in Great Britain. It is slightly constipating.

5.2 Clinical Use

Dihydrocodeine is used in the rheumatic disorders as an analgesic with mild sedative and constipating properties. It is much more effective given by intramuscular injection when it is considered to be potentially addictive.

5.3 Preparations and Dosage

Tablets of dihydrocodeine tartrate 30mg; 1 to 2 as required, or as a sterile solution 50mg of dihydrocodeine tartrate in 1ml with 0.1% of sodium metabisulphite for intramuscular injection. An elixir (syrup) containing 10mg per 5ml is also available in some countries.

5.4 Cautions

Use with caution in patients with constipation, asthma or liver disease. There is a risk of addiction with parenteral administration. Dihydrocodeine should therefore not be used intramuscularly in individuals considered to be potential addicts.

6. Analgesic Addictive Drugs

These analgesics are never used unless the prognosis is grave and pain is rendering reasonable life impossible. Such conditions are malignant disease of bone or joint or advanced rheumatoid disease in extremis and associated with great pain. In such cases the following strong analgesics may be useful:

6.1 Dipipanone

Dipipanone, 4,4-diphenyl-6-piperidino-heptan-3-one hydrochloride monohydrate, has a strong analgesic action which begins about 15 minutes after an intramuscular injection and lasts for 4 to 6 hours. Given alone it has relatively little hypnotic or sedative action but 10mg dipipanone hydrochloride mixed with 30mg cyclizine hydrochloride may be given by mouth in tablet form with considerable effect 6 to 12-hourly. Its action may be prolonged in the presence of severe renal or hepatic disease.

6.2 Morphine or Diamorphine (heroin)

Morphine or diamorphine may be given orally with alcohol and sometimes cocaine (10mg) in small doses of 5 to 15mg in terminal cases every 3 to 6 hours to anticipate rather than to treat severe pain as it arises, increasing dosage as found necessary. A phenothiazine, such as chlorpromazine or prochlorperazine can be added if nausea, vomiting or agitation occurs. Such elixirs have a shelf-life of about 3 weeks and should be used within this time or discarded. Diamorphine and cocaine elixir, BPC (1973) is:

Diamorphine hydrochloride 1g
Cocaine hydrochloride 1g
Alcohol (90%) 125ml
Syrup 250ml
Chloroform water to 1,000ml

The use of cocaine is considered questionable by many. It is not truly euphorious or antidepressive and may cause nightmares, mental confusion and occasionally excitement. Morphine can replace diamorphine while chlorpromazine elixir, BPC (1973) can replace the simple syrup if required.

Dosage starts with 2.5 to 5mg diamorphine and 3.75 to 7.5mg morphine, 3 to 6-hourly; initial dosage being doubled if found to be inadequate. Thereafter, dose increments and spacing depends on the individual case. In many cases, such a programme of oral medication is adequate with injections of morphine or diamorphine only required terminally or not at all. It must be emphasised that this programme is only for the terminal case with an extremely bad prognosis. The effectiveness of morphine: diamorphine orally would seem to be about 1:1.5, but Twycross (1976) considers there is little clinical difference between the analgesics used in this way.

6.3 Levorphanol

Levorphanol tartrate is the dihydrate of (-)-3-hydroxy-N-methylmorphinan hydrogen tartrate. It has the actions and uses, therapeutic and undesirable, of morphine but is almost as effective by mouth as by injection. By mouth, dosage is 1.5 to 4.5mg (1 to 3 tablets of 1.5mg). The subcutaneous and intramuscular dose is 2 to 4mg. It should not be given with alcohol.

References and Recommended Reading

Editorial: Dangers of dextropropoxyphene. British Medical Journal 1: 668 (1977).

Loan, W.B. and Morrison, J.D.: Strong analgesics: pharmacological and therapeutic aspects. Drugs 5: 108 (1973).

Parkhouse, J.: Simple analgesics. Drugs 10: 366 (1975).

Twycross, R.G.: The measurement of pain in terminal carcinoma. Journal of International Medical Research 4 (Suppl. 2): 58 (1976).

Whittington, R.M.: Dextropropoxyphene (Distalgesic) overdosage in the West Midlands. British Medical Journal 2: 172 (1977).

Chapter VII

Drugs Used in the Control of Gout

1. Colchicine

Colchicum has long been used as a remedy for gout, whereas the aklaloid colchicine, was isolated from the root of the autumn crocus, *Colchicum autumnale,* in 1820.

1.1 Actions

Colchicine is an anti-inflammatory and antimitotic agent which acts by interfering with leucocyte responses (Malawista, 1968). In acute gout, it inhibits leucocyte migration and interrupts the inflammatory response to urate crystal formation by reducing phagocytosis. The reduced metabolic activity of the leucocyte results in less local lactic acid formation, resulting in a reduced tendency to urate crystal formation and a lessened inflammatory response. Colchicine also interferes with the formation of kinins. While colchicine is chiefly of value in acute gout, some response has also been reported in the arthritis associated with sarcoidosis, erythema nodosum and calcium pyrophosphate crystal formation. It has no effect upon urate metabolism or the concentration of urate in the serum or urine.

1.2 Absorption, Distribution and Elimination

Oral absorption of colchicine is rapid. After intravenous administration, colchicine leaves the blood rapidly (plasma half-life 0.32 hours) and is widely distributed. It is concentrated in the kidney, liver, spleen and intestinal tract and has been demonstrated to be present in leucocytes 10 days after administration of a single dose. The apparent volume of distribution is greater than the total body weight, averaging 1.1L/kg (Ertel et al., 1976). It is partly deacetylated in the liver, and the greater part of both colchicine and its metabolites is excreted in the bile and intestinal secretions. However, up to 20% is excreted in the urine unchanged where it has been demonstrated to be present for up to 10 days after a single intravenous dose (Wallace, 1974). In renal failure, there is a reduction in the rate of renal excretion of colchicine, but there is no need to modify dosage when used short-term in acute gout.

1.3 Side-effects

Adverse reactions to colchicine are usually dose-related and occur primarily due to overdosage. The first symptom is usually diarrhoea with some abdominal pain, although occasional patients develop nausea and vomiting before the diarrhoea. High dosage colchicine therapy can lead to malabsorption with mild steatorrhoea and malabsorption of vitamin B_{12}, whereas gross overdosage results in a haemorrhagic gastroenteritis and damage to many tissues. With usual therapeutic doses, diarrhoea or nausea is the only significant complication.

Because of its antimitotic effect, damage to the bone marrow during colchicine therapy has been anticipated, but this is rarely seen with the use of dosages which are therapeutically effective. Prolonged use has no apparent toxic effect upon testicular function (Bremner and Paulsen, 1976). Alopecia and myopathy have been reported with prolonged usage, but must be rare.

1.4 Clinical Use and Dosage

If colchicine is to be used in the acute attack of gout, it should be used early in the attack. The initial dose should be 1mg orally, followed by 0.5mg 2-hourly until gastrointestinal toxicity (usually diarrhoea or vomiting) occurs or the pain is relieved. Between 4 and 8mg of colchicine will usually be required. As the effective dose in acute gouty arthritis is close to the toxic dose, most patients being treated for acute gout with colchicine for the first time will develop some diarrhoea and this is the sign to withhold further colchicine.

The dose which produces diarrhoea remains reasonably constant for any individual, so that, if colchicine is used on the second occasion for acute gout, the total dose of colchicine administered can be limited to 0.5mg less than the dose which previously caused diarrhoea. Colchicine is effective in up to 90% of patients with acute gouty arthritis, although relief may not be complete until 24 hours after cessation of treatment or the development of gastrointestinal toxicity. If an intravenous preparation is available, colchicine can be given in a single dose of 2mg well diluted in 20ml of saline. Systemic side-effects from this are rare, although any local extravasation may produce a slough. The lower dosage range of colchicine should be used in patients with severe renal or hepatic failure.

Colchicine in low dosage is also an effective prophylactic agent against acute attacks of gouty arthritis (Yu and Gutman, 1961). Such regular prophylactic use of colchicine will be associated with fewer acute attacks in patients either with recurrent gouty arthritis or numerous low grade attacks, at times when surgery is undertaken and during institution of urate-lowering therapy. Its effectiveness is unrelated to whether patients are hyperuricaemic or normouricaemic.

The prophylactic dose will vary between 0.5 and 1.5mg daily, although 0.5mg twice daily is usually satisfactory. The prophylactic dose should be adjusted so as to cause no side-effects and should be continued for at least 12 months after the last acute attack in gout. Prophylactic dosage should be reduced in patients with severe renal or hepatic failure.

The manifestations of familial Mediterranean fever (recurrent polyserositis) can be suppressed by the daily administration of between 1 and 1.5mg of colchicine (Goldfinger, 1972). This genetic condition often manifests as pleuritic lesions or arthritis affecting one or more of the large joints.

1.5 Preparations

Colchicine is available as a tablet of 0.5mg (deteriorates in light). An intravenous preparation (0.5mg in 1ml) is sometimes available.

1.6 Cautions

Use with caution in patients with impaired cardiac, renal or hepatic function. Gastrointestinal symptoms are more likely to occur in patients with peptic ulcer or diseases of the colon. Colchicine is contraindicated in pregnancy.

2. Probenecid

2.1 Actions

Probenecid, p-(di-n-propylsulfamyl) benzoic acid, the first clinically useful uricosuric agent, lowers the serum urate by promoting its renal elimination (Klippen et al., 1974). It acts as a competitive inhibitor of the renal tubular mechanism for reabsorption of urate (fig. 1). Probenecid also inhibits the renal tubular secretion of penicillin, the property for which it was first used; it is also said to block the transport of serotonin and dopamine out of the cerebrospinal fluid.

2.2 Absorption, Distribution and Elimination

Probenecid is readily absorbed from the alimentary tract and about 90% is rapidly bound to plasma proteins. It has a low volume of distribution of 0.12 to 0.18L/kg. Its distribution, therefore, is largely confined to the extracellular fluid. It

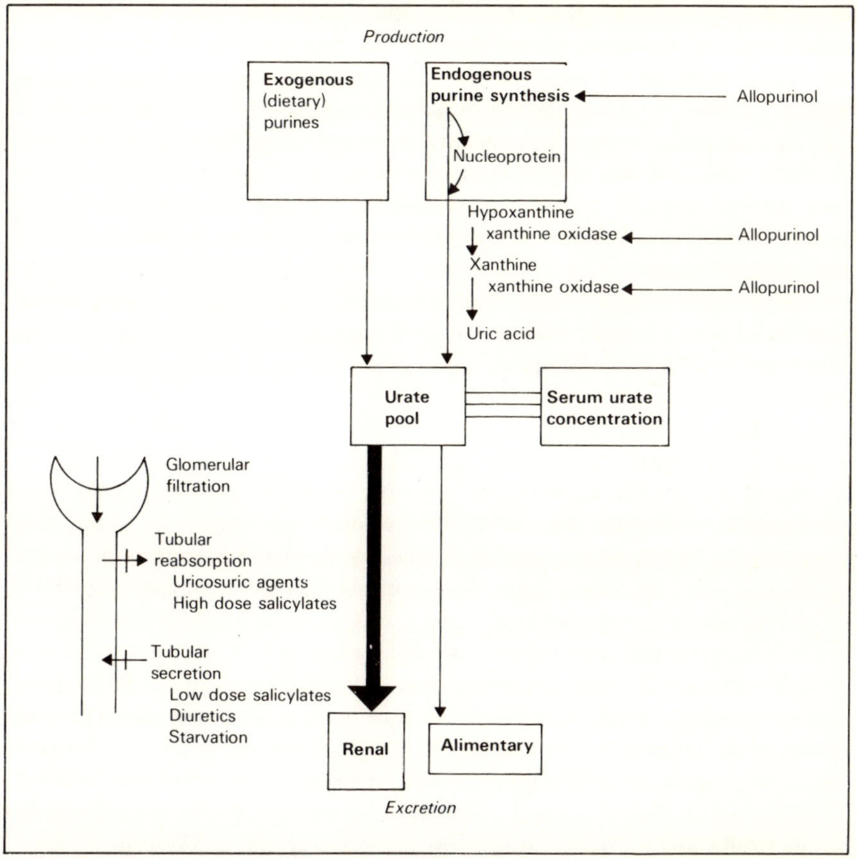

Fig. 1. Schematic representation of the urate pool (a balance between urate production and excretion) and its modification by urate-altering drugs [from Hart in Avery (Ed) Drug Treatment, p.650, ADIS Press, Sydney 1976; by permission].

has a plasma half-life of between 4 and 12 hours, depending on dosage. At least 80% of the administered dose of probenecid is rapidly metabolised in the liver either to its acyl-monoglucuronide or by oxidation at a variety of positions on its n-propyl side chain (Dayton and Perel, 1971). It is likely that the metabolites are also uricosuric. Excretion is by the renal route.

2.3 Drug Interactions

Aspirin in low doses blocks the uricosuric action of probenecid and probenecid also reduces the renal excretion of salicylates. Probenecid also inhibits the renal tubular secretion of a variety of weak organic acids, particularly penicillin, ampicillin, cephalothin (but not cephaloridine), dapsone and salicylates, as well as pantothenic acid, androsterone and di-iodotyrosine. This competition between drugs for renal tubular secretion is used to therapeutic advantage when probenecid is given to increase serum levels of penicillins by delaying their renal excretion.

Probenecid prolongs the half-life and increases the serum concentration of indomethacin and metabolites due to impairment of its renal excretion, but whether reduced doses of indomethacin are needed is not clear (see chapt. II; sect. 4.3). It also inhibits the conjugation of benzoic acid derivatives with glycine. Probenecid prolongs the half-life and increases serum concentrations of rifampicin, probably by impairment of its hepatic uptake, but there is little justification for use of probenecid to reduce the usual dose of rifampicin.

2.4 Side-effects

Up to 8 % of patients are reported to suffer from gastric irritation after use of probenecid (Gutman and Yu, 1957), chiefly when large doses are given. Such symptoms can sometimes be modified by adjusting the time relationships of the dose or its relationship with meals. Up to 5 % of patients show signs of hypersensitivity or a rash. Serious side-effects are rare.

Use of probenecid will precipitate an acute attack in a significant proportion of patients with gouty arthritis. Colchicine, given in the prophylactic dose of 0.5mg once or twice daily, will reduce this tendency. Because of the associated increased renal excretion of urate, particularly during the early stages of therapy, the use of probenecid should be accompanied by the induction of a persistent water diuresis and/or alkalinisation of urine. This is aimed at minimising the risk of uric acid crystal deposition within tubules and collecting ducts or the formation of uric acid calculi.

2.5 Clinical Use

As the increase in urinary excretion of urate is greater during the early stages of therapy, it is wise for the initial dose to be small and for increments in dosage to be gradual. The risk of uric acid crystal formation in the urine is minimised by the promotion of a water diuresis. Alkalinisation of urine is desirable in the first few weeks of therapy when the uricosuria is greatest. Once the serum urate has stabilised at a lower level within the normal range, the intense uricosuria subsides, although the total 24 hour excretion of uric acid on probenecid therapy is greater than that prior to its administration. However, such as increase is relatively insignificant in comparison with other factors which cause fluctuation in the urine urate, particularly variation in dietary purine consumption. It is nonetheless mandatory always to maintain a good urine volume during uricosuric therapy, exceeding 2 litres per 24 hours at the very least.

The uricosuric effect of probenecid falls with impairment of glomerular filtration rate and very little uricosuric response can be detected at creatinine clearances of less than about 50 to 70ml/min. Above this level, however, an increased dose of probenecid may still result in a uricosuric response.

2.6 Preparations and Dosage

Probenecid is available in 500mg tablets; the more recent film-coated preparations have been associated with a lower incidence of nausea. Very low dosage may retain urate in some subjects (Yu and Gutman, 1955) and the usual uricosuric dose will vary between 1 and 3g per day, given in 2 to 3 divided doses; 1.5 to 2g per day is effective in most patients.

2.7 Cautions

Aspirin should be avoided in patients receiving probenecid. Because of the risk of uric acid crystal formation, particular caution is needed in the very frequent patients with habitually poor urine volumes. Probenecid is contraindicated in: (a) patients with urate overproduction and hence a high urinary uric acid excretion; (b) patients with a past history of renal calculus of any type; (c) patients with a persistently poor urine volume; (d) hypersensitivity to probenecid. Treatment should not commence during an acute attack of gout.

3. Sulphinpyrazone

3.1 Actions

Sulphinpyrazone, 1,2-diphenyl-4-(2-phenylsulfinethyl)-3,5 pyrazolidinendione, like phenylbutazone is a pyrazolone derivative. Whereas phenylbutazone has a strong anti-inflammatory action but a mild uricosuric action (chapt. II; sect. 2.1), sulphinpyrazone has a very mild anti-inflammatory action but a very potent uricosuric action (Emmerson, 1963). On a weight-for-weight basis, it is between 3 and 6 times more potent as a uricosuric than probenecid (fig. 2).

Sulphinpyrazone has been shown to reduce platelet aggregation and adhesiveness and to prolong platelet survival (Smythe et al., 1965). It inhibits the platelet response to stimuli which cause the loss from the platelet of ADP and other biologically active materials essential for platelet aggregation and thrombus formation. Thus, it has been used with some benefit in patients with embolisation from prosthetic heart valves, rheumatic heart disease, recurrent venous thromboses and thromboses of arterio-venous shunts.

3.2 Absorption, Distribution and Elimination

Sulphinpyrazone is rapidly and completely absorbed from the alimentary tract with a peak serum concentration within 1 to 2 hours. Its plasma half-life is between 2 and 4 hours. It is very strongly protein bound (98 %) and its distribution is thus confined to the extracellular fluid. Only a small proportion of the drug in the plasma is in the metabolised form. Para-hydroxylated metabolites are formed in the liver, and these are also uricosuric in man. Excretion is rapid and complete, the largest proportion of a single dose being excreted in the first 6 hours (Dieterle et al., 1975). Within 4 days after a single dose, 85 % can be recovered from the urine and 10 % from the faeces. Of the amount recovered from the urine, 50 % is as the unchanged drug, 9 % as the parahydroxymetabolite, 3 % as a sulphone metabolite and 1 % as the 4-hy-

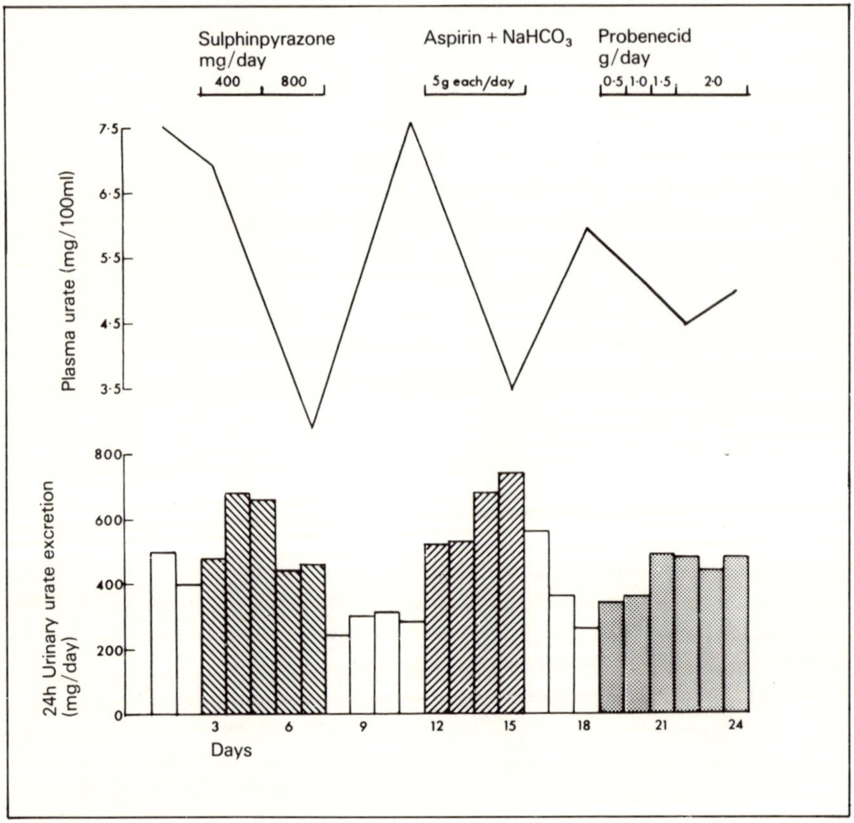

Fig. 2. The effect on the plasma urate concentration and the urinary urate excretion of doses of sulphinpyrazone (400 and 800mg/day), aspirin and sodium bicarbonate (5g of each/day), probenecid (0.5, 1.0, 1.5 and 2.0g/day).

droxy metabolite. 30 % can be recovered as a glucuronide complex. The plasma half-life is prolonged in renal failure.

3.3 Drug Interactions

As with probenecid, low doses of aspirin block the uricosuric effect of sulphinpyrazone and sulphinpyrazone blocks the uricosuric effect of salicylates (Yu et al., 1963). Probenecid markedly inhibits the renal excretion of sulphinpyrazone and its metabolites (Perel et al., 1969).

3.4 Side-effects

Between 10 and 15 % of patients suffer from gastrointestinal symptoms, chiefly nausea, and this is somewhat more common than with probenecid. Sulphinpyrazone may also aggravate or reactivate peptic ulcers. As it is a pyrazole derivative, one is cautious about its potential for bone marrow depression. However, extensive clinical use has shown this to be a very rare association and much less common than occurs with phenylbutazone (chapt. II; sect. 2.4).

The risk of uric acid stone formation exists as with probenecid (section 2.4, 2.5), but because of its more potent uricosuric action, the risk of uric acid crystal formation within the renal tract might be expected to be greater. Hence, the greater importance of maintaining a consistent large volume of urine (preferably exceeding 3 litres/day) which should be alkalinised during the early stages of treatment. It is wise to avoid intermittent therapy which will cause fluctuation in the serum urate and the intermittent risks to the kidney of intense uricosuria.

3.5 Clinical Use

Regular treatment with sulphinpyrazone will restore a normal serum urate and if this is maintained for a sufficient period, it will prevent recurrent attacks of acute gouty arthritis. As vascular disease has been found in a significant proportion of patients with gout, the action of sulphinpyrazone in reducing platelet adhesiveness and aggregation may be beneficial to such patients, although no controlled studies have yet been undertaken. The uricosuric effect is reduced in renal insufficiency and is negligible at a creatinine clearance of less than 50ml/min. Above such a value, however, an increased dose of sulphinpyrazone may often maintain a useful increase in urinary urate excretion in patients who are unable to tolerate other drugs.

3.6 Preparations and Dosage

Sulphinpyrazone is stable at room temperature and is available in 100mg tablets. A uricosuric effect can usually be achieved at between 200 and 400mg per day which, despite the relatively short plasma half-life, can be clinically effective if given in two divided doses per day. The dose can be increased to 800mg per day if an insufficient response occurs at the lower dose range. Care concerning the maintenance of a large urine volume is mandatory.

3.7 Cautions

Aspirin therapy should be avoided in patients receiving sulphinpyrazone and the risk of uric acid crystal formation in the renal tract must likewise be minimised. Sulphinpyrazone is contraindicated in: (a) urate overproducers who would already be at an increased risk of urate calculi; (b) gouty nephropathy of significant degree; (c) patients with renal calculi, whether due to urate or of other varieties; or (d) hypersensitivity to sulphinpyrazone, severe hepatic or renal disease. Treatment should not commence during an acute attack of gout.

4. Allopurinol

Allopurinol, 4-hydroxypyrazolo-(3,4-d)-pyrimidine, an isomer of hypoxanthine, was synthesised in 1956.

4.1 Actions

Allopurinol acts as an inhibitor of xanthine oxidase which, in man, it inhibits to approximately 50%. Xanthine oxidase catalyses the conversion of hypoxanthine to xanthine and of xanthine to uric acid, so that inhibition of xanthine oxidase will lead to both a reduction in the amount of hypoxanthine and xanthine (fig. 1). Thus, during the use of allopurinol, the concentration of uric acid in both serum and urine will fall and the concentration of hypoxanthine and of xanthine in both serum and urine will rise (fig. 3). Of these, xanthine is less soluble than uric acid, but the redistribution of purine excretion among three substances minimises the risk of crystallisation of the increased amounts of xanthine which are produced. The xanthine and hypoxanthine (oxypurines) are readily excreted by the kidney. Following oral administration, there is a fall in the uric acid content of both plasma and urine within 24 to 48 hours. Withdrawal of allopurinol results in a return towards normal values within a few days, although some of the other metabolic effects may still be detected between 7 and 10 days after withdrawal of the drug.

As well as diversion of purine end products from uric acid to xanthine and hypoxanthine, the administration of allopurinol results in a reduction in total purine production. Failure to observe such an effect occurs chiefly in subjects with a deficiency of the enzyme, hypoxanthine guanine phosphoribosyl-transferase (HGPRT), which promotes reutilisation of the purine bases. This reduction in total purine syn-

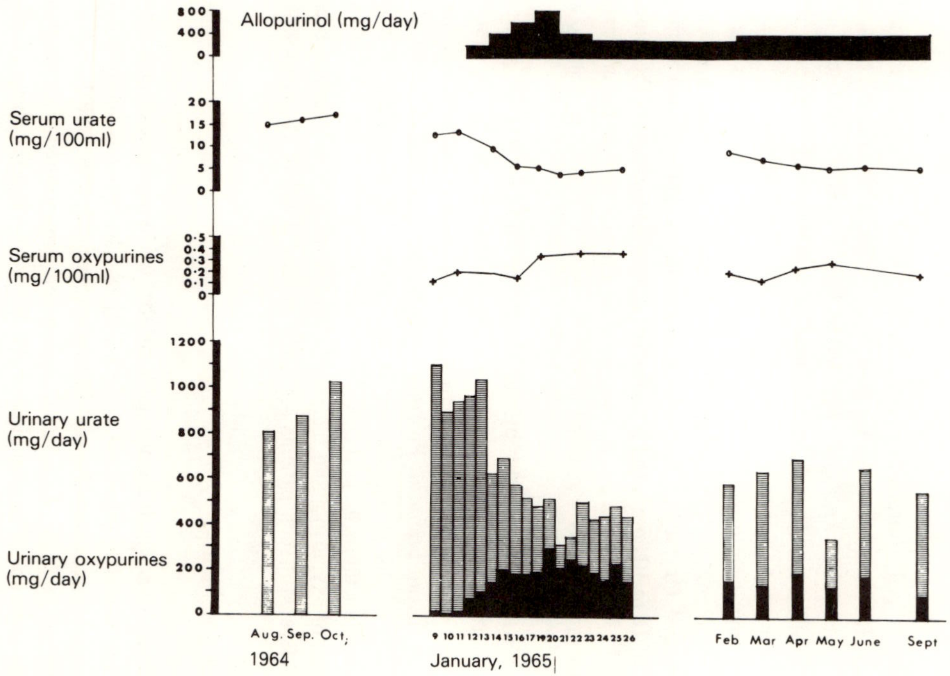

Fig. 3. The effect of allopurinol in a patient with the urate overproduction of polycythaemia vera. This shows the effect of various doses on the serum concentrations and urinary excretions of urate and the oxypurines, xanthine and hypoxanthine (from Emmerson: Aust. Ann. Med. 16: 205-214, 1967; by permission).

thesis is due principally to the utilisation of phosphoribosylpyrophosphate (PRPP) by allopurinol in its conversion to allopurinol ribonucleotide. This causes a reduced concentration of PRPP in red cells and in other tissues and the reduced PRPP availability results in reduced *de novo* purine biosynthesis.

4.2 Absorption, Distribution and Elimination

Allopurinol is well absorbed from the alimentary tract and has a plasma half-life of 2 to 8 hours. It is a substrate for (as well as an inhibitor of) xanthine oxidase, so that much of it (about 60 %) is rapidly oxidised by hepatic xanthine oxidase to its major active metabolite, oxypurinol, an analogue of xanthine. The remainder of the allopurinol which is not oxidised to oxypurinol is converted to allopurinol ribonucleoside and allopurinol ribonucleotide. Some of the oxypurinol produced is also converted to the corresponding ribonucleoside and ribonucleotide, although much of it remains unchanged. Oxypurinol has a much longer plasma half-life than allopurinol (of ther order of 18 to 30 hours) and is probably responsible for most of the inhibition of xanthine oxidase which occurs *in vivo*. Both allopurinol and oxypurinol are distributed evenly in total body water and neither is bound to plasma proteins to a significant degree.

Allopurinol is cleared rapidly by the kidney, probably largely by glomerular filtration. Oxypurinol is filtered at the glomerulus and reabsorbed by the tubules so that it is excreted much more slowly than allopurinol and its renal handling appears to be similar to that of uric acid. Probenecid accelerates the renal excretion of oxypurinol and this results in a reduction in the efficacy of allopurinol if it is administered in conjunction with probenecid. In renal insufficiency, there is a reduction in the clearance of oxypurinol and the plasma concentration of oxypurinol becomes considerably elevated if such patients are given normal doses of allopurinol.

4.3 Drug Interactions

The effect of drugs which are normally metabolised by xanthine oxidase is potentiated by the concurrent administration of allopurinol. The two most important drugs in this group are 6-mercaptopurine and its precursor azathioprine, the dose of which should be reduced to 25 % of the usual dose when administered with allopurinol. There is some evidence of potentiation of the action of cytotoxic drugs, especially cyclophosphamide, when given with allopurinol, although the mechanism by which this occurs is not understood (cyclophosphamide is not metabolised by xanthine oxidase). Nonetheless, there appears to be an increased risk of bone marrow depression if allopurinol is administered with cyclophosphamide.

An increased incidence of skin rash has been reported in patients receiving ampicillin simultaneously with allopurinol.

Allopurinol has also been reported to prolong the half-life of drugs which are metabolised by the hepatic microsomal enzyme oxidising system, thus leading to possible potentiation of effect (Vessell et al., 1970). This appears to apply to dicoumarol, but the clinical significance of this observation is not yet established. Allopurinol does not alter warfarin metabolism. Prolongation by allopurinol of the half-life of probenecid has been reported (Tjandramaga and Cucinell, 1971), but this is of doubtful significance. Similarly, marked prolongation of the half-life of chlorpropamide has been reported in some, but not all, patients also treated with allopurinol.

4.4 Side-effects

Serious complications of allopurinol therapy have been uncommon in over 10 years of clinical use, the most common being a rash which occurs in up to 4% of patients. In the presence of renal insufficiency, however, the incidence of skin reactions may rise to about 15% (Frisch et al., 1974); dosage should be reduced in patients with impaired renal function. In 10% of patients with a rash, this may be associated with severe systemic manifestations such as fever, eosinophilia and serious hypersensitivity (Kantor, 1970; Mills, 1971). Gastric intolerance is not infrequently seen but this is rarely serious and can be minimised by administering tablets after meals.

Other reactions, such as vasculitis, hepatitis, leucopenia and thrombocytopenia have been seen, but rarely, and their importance and frequency is difficult to interpret. Crystals of xanthine, hypoxanthine and oxypurinol have been noted in the skeletal muscles of gouty patients treated with allopurinol but this is of doubtful clinical significance because uric acid crystals have also been demonstrated by this technique in untreated gouty patients (Watts et al., 1971). As already mentioned (section 4.1), allopurinol decreases intracellular PRPP. Another biochemical observation is the partial inhibition of pyramidine biosynthesis by allopurinol leading to orotidinuria and orotic aciduria (Fox et al., 1970). It appears not to have clinical significance.

Oxypurinol stones have been reported after very large oral dosage with oxypurinol (but not with allopurinol). There is no evidence of incorporation of allopurinol into nucleic acids (Nelson and Elion, 1975).

4.5 Clinical Use

Reduction of serum and urine urate excretion by allopurinol is particularly indicated in patients with hyperuricaemia and gout due to urate over production, whether of primary origin (as in HGRPT deficiency) or secondary to marrow proliferation as in myeloproliferative disorders (fig. 4). It can prevent the tendency to uric acid nephropathy which is frequently associated with such conditions.

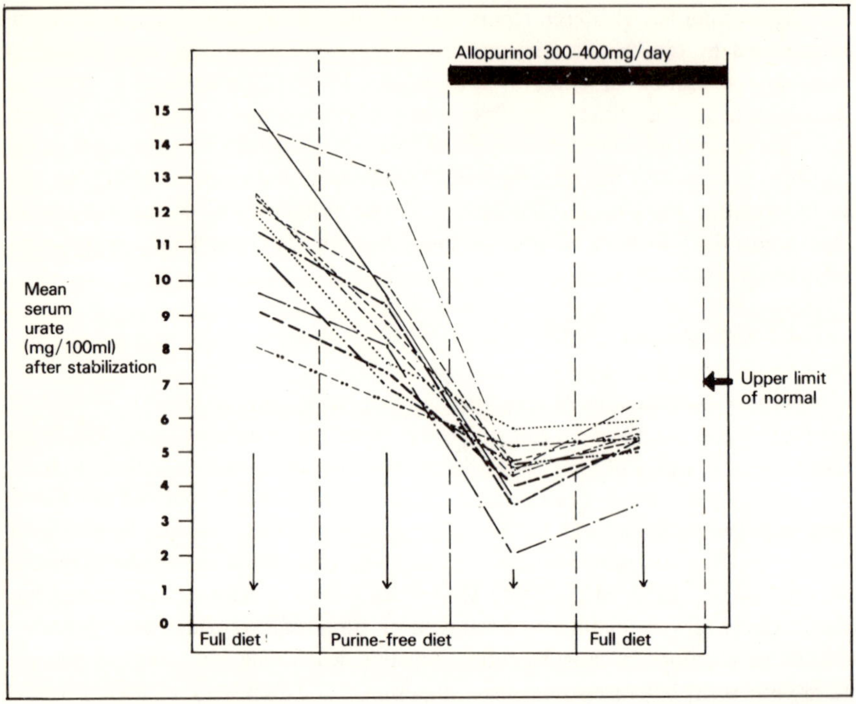

Fig. 4. The effect of allopurinol on the serum urate concentrations of patients with gout after stabilisation on purine-containing and purine-free diets (from Emmerson: Aust. Ann. Med. 16: 205-214, 1967; by permission).

Allopurinol is of particular value when gout is associated with renal disease or in the presence of uric acid stones. There is suggestive evidence that allopurinol may also minimise the development of stones which do not primarily consist of uric acid (Smith and Boyce, 1969) such as calcium oxalate (Coe and Kavalach, 1974).

4.6 Preparations and Dosage

Allopurinol is available as 100 and 300mg tablets. A normal serum urate concentration can be achieved in most patients with a daily dose between 100 and 300mg. Because of the long plasma half-life of oxypurinol, the active metabolite of allopurinol, a single daily dose of allopurinol may well be as effective as a divided dose regimen. A single daily dose of 300mg each morning is now commonly used. If hyperuricaemia is not controlled by this regimen, the dose could be increased to between 400 and 600mg daily but a higher dose than this should be used only if all other factors promoting hyperuricaemia have been corrected. Lowering of the serum urate by allopurinol can result in precipitation of acute attacks of gout. The tendency for this to occur can be minimised by prophylactic colchicine therapy and by ensuring that any changes in serum urate concentration are gradual.

4.7 Cautions

Provided due allowance is made for side-effects and interactions with other drugs (see section 4.3, 4.4), the main reasons for caution in the use of allopurinol would be in patients with gross overproduction of urate (such as the Lesch-Nyhan syndrome) in whom there is a potential risk of xanthine calculi or of xanthine nephropathy if urine volume is poor. It is important that the dose be kept to a minimum in patients with renal disease, due to the decreased rate of elimination of oxypurinol, the active metabolite of allopurinol (see section 4.2).

References and Recommended Reading

Colchicine

Bremner, W.J. and Paulsen, C.A.: Colchicine and testicular function in man. New England Journal of Medicine 294: 1384 (1976).

Ertel, N.H.; Mittler, J.C.; Akgun, S. and Wallace, S.L.: Radioimmunoassay for colchicine in plasma and urine. Science 193: 233 (1976).

Goldfinger, S.E.: Colchicine for familial Mediterranean fever. New England Journal of Medicine 287: 1302 (1972).

Malawista, S.E.: Colchicine: A common mechanism for the anti-inflammatory and anti-mitotic effects. Arthritis and Rheumatism 11: 191 (1968).

Wallace, S.L.: Colchicine. Seminars in Arthritis and Rheumatism 3: 369 (1974).

Yu, T-F. and Gutman, A.B.: Efficacy of colchicine prophylaxis in gout. Annals of Internal Medicine 55: 179 (1961).

Probenecid

Dayton, P.G. and Perel, J.M.: The metabolism of probenecid in man. Annals of the New York Academy of Science 179: 399 (1971).

Gutman, A.B. and Yu, T-F.: Protracted uricosuric therapy in tophaceous gout. Lancet 2: 1256 (1957).

Kippen, I.; Whitehouse, M.W. and Klinenberg, M.W.: Pharmacology of uricosuric drugs. Annals of the Rheumatic Diseases 33: 391 (1974).

Yu, T-F. and Gutman, A.B.: Paradoxical retention of uric acid by uricosuric drugs in low dosage. Proceedings of the Society for Experimental Biology and Medicine (New York) 90: 542 (1955).

Sulphinpyrazone

Dieterle, W.; Faigle, J.W.; Mory, H.; Richter, W.J. and Theobald, W.: Biotransformation and pharmacokinetics of sulphinpyrazone in man. Clinical Pharmacology 9: 135 (1975).

Emmerson, B.T.: A comparison of uricosuric agents in gout with special reference to sulphinpyrazone. Medical Journal of Australia 1: 839 (1963).

Perel, J.M.; Dayton, P.G.; Snell, M.M.; Yu, T-F. and Gutman, A.B.: Studies of interactions among drugs in man at the renal level: Probenecid and sulphinpyrazone. Clinical Pharmacology and Therapeutics 10: 834 (1969).

Smythe, H.A.; Ogryzlo, M.A.; Murphy, E.A. and Mustard, J.F.: The effect of sulphinpyrazone (Anurane) on platelet economy and blood coagulation in man. Canadian Medical Association Journal 92: 818 (1965).

Yu, T-F.; Dayton, P.G. and Gutman, A.B.: Mutual suppression of the uricosuric effects of sulfinpyrazone and salicylate: A study in interactions between drugs. Journal of Clinical Investigation 42: 1330 (1963).

Allopurinol

Coe, F.L. and Kavalach, A.G.: Hypercalciuria and hyperuricosuria in patients with calcium nephrolithiasis. New England Journal of Medicine 291: 1344 (1974).

Fox, R.M.; Royce-Smith, D. and O'Sullivan, W.J.: Orotidinuria induced by allopurinol. Science 168: 861 (1970).

Frisch, J.M.; Lovatt, G.E.; Sproit, A.R.M. and Turmer, P.: The Adverse Reaction Profile of Allopurinol. Proceedings of the 12th International Congress of Internal Medicine 412-419 (1974).

Kantor, G.L.: Toxic epidermal necrolysis, azotemia and death after allopurinol therapy. Journal of the American Medical Association 212: 478 (1970).

Kelley, W.N.: Effects of drugs on uric acid in man. Annual Review of Pharmacology 15: 327 (1975).

Mills, R.M.: Severe hypersensitivity reactions associated with allopurinol. Journal of the American Medical Association 216: 799 (1971).

Nelson, D.J. and Elion, G.B.: Metabolism of (6-^{14}C) allopurinol — Lack of incorporation of allopurinol into nucleic acids. Biochemical Pharmacology 24: 1235 (1975).

Smith, M.J.V. and Boyce, W.H.: Allopurinol and urolithiasis. Journal of Urology 102: 750 (1969).

Tjandramaga, T.B. and Cucinell, S.A.: Interaction of probenecid and allopurinol in gouty subjects. Federation Proceedings 30: 392, Abstract 1112 (1971).

Vesell, E.S. : Passananti, G.T. and Greene, F.E.: Impairment of drug metabolism in man by allopurinol and nortriptyline. New England Journal of Medicine 283: 1484 (1970).

Watts, R.W.E. : Scott, J.T.; Chalmers, R.A.; Bitensky, L. and Chayen, J.: Microscopic studies on skeletal muscle in gout patients treated with allopurinol. Quarterly Journal of Medicine 40: 1 (1971).

Chapter VIII

Rheumatoid Arthritis

Drug treatment is only a part of the total management of rheumatoid arthritis. It is nevertheless an important part. The clinician who makes a diagnosis of rheumatoid arthritis may pause to explain the disease, outline a plan of treatment and make light of the prognosis, but before long he will surely take out his pen and write a prescription. But what for? The number of available drugs has risen greatly in recent years and it is increasingly important for the clinician to have some plan if he is to avoid selecting drugs at random.

The fundamental premise of the treatment plan is recognition of two entirely different types of drug therapy: (1) drugs which simply relieve symptoms, non-specific or symptomatic therapy; and (2) specific drugs such as gold and penicillamine, which act slowly in an unknown way on the rheumatoid disease process, and given long-term, appear to alter the course of persistently active or progressive disease. Drugs for symptomatic therapy include simple analgesics, non-steroidal anti-inflammatory analgesics and corticosteroids (chapters II, IV, VI). Simple analgesics and non-steroidal anti-inflammatory analgesics represent the first step in the treatment of rheumatoid arthritis. The aim of the first step is to find the drug regimen which provides optimum effectiveness with the lowest incidence of side-effects.

1. The First Step — Early Active Disease

The order of use of non-specific or symptomatic remedies is discussed in chapter I (sect. 3). The traditional view is that aspirin is the first line treatment of rheumatoid arthritis and that the newer drugs should be used when it fails, usually as a result of side-effects. This view is supported by the low cost of aspirin and by its antiquity — the side-effects and problems are at least well known. The alternative view is that it is better to use safer and better tolerated drugs first, even if they are less effective. The more effective propionic acid derivatives such as naproxen and fenoprofen (see chapter II), have been shown to be as effective as full doses of aspirin and with a strikingly lower incidence of side-effects (Huskisson et al., 1974). These drugs therefore make a strong claim to replace aspirin as the first line of therapy. Not only do they cause less side-effects, but more patients are able to continue to take them. There is a striking individual variation in response, so that some patients like one drug, some like another (Huskisson et al., 1976). If the propionic acid derivatives are considered as a group of drugs, and if the clinician is prepared to try them all to find the best one for each patient, the group has a major advantage over aspirin. It should be possible to maintain at least two-thirds of all patients with rheumatoid arthritis on one of the propionic acid derivatives which is both effective and well tolerated. This group of drugs therefore represents an alternative first line of therapy to aspirin.

There are now a number of other non-steroidal anti-inflammatory analgesics which also have advantages over aspirin in the incidence of side-effects. Such drugs include tolmetin, azapropazone and sulindac. They could also be used first, or as an alternative to propionic acid derivatives in patients who fail to respond or who develop side-effects. All these drugs are much more expensive than aspirin, so that some patients may prefer to try aspirin first. There are also many different ways of taking aspirin (Huskisson, 1974; Medical Letter, 1974) and many 'sophisticated' preparations reduce the incidence of occult gastrointestinal bleeding and gastric side-effects. They include buffered, enteric-coated and microencapsulated preparations. These 'sophisticated' formulations cost much more than plain or soluble aspirin so that much of the advantage of the cheapness of aspirin is lost.

The advantage of starting with propionic acid derivatives or other less toxic drugs is well illustrated with a drug like phenylbutazone. Phenylbutazone is a very effective anti-inflammatory agent but causes gastric side-effects and rarely fatal aplastic anaemia. It also has a marked potential for interaction with important groups of drugs which might be given concurrently (see chapter II; sect. 2.3, 2.4). No-one would deny the value of phenylbutazone in selected cases but it is better to use a safer drug if possible. Using a 'safety-first' philosophy, patients will only receive phenylbutazone when they have failed to respond to simpler safer remedies.

Indomethacin, like aspirin and phenylbutazone, causes more side-effects than the propionic acid derivatives and is therefore best reserved for patients who fail to respond to them. There is, however, one special use for indomethacin in rheumatoid arthritis. When given in a large dose at night, indomethacin is particularly effective in relieving night pain, improving sleep and reducing the duration of morning stiffness (Huskisson, 1976). Patients can often tolerate 75 to 100mg at night without side-effects when the same dose in the day produces headaches or gastric disturbance. Presumably, the side-effects occur while the patient is asleep. This dose can be given as a suppository (100mg) but the same dose by mouth is equally effective and often preferred.

Regular day-time anti-inflammatory therapy, with naproxen for example, can usefully be combined with indomethacin at night in patients with night pain or morning stiffness. Some other anti-inflammatory drugs such as ketoprofen or naproxen in twice normal dosage on retiring can be used as an alternative to indomethacin at night. Apart from this combination, there seems little point in combining anti-inflammatory drugs. Thus, aspirin was shown to be no more effective (and no less effective) when given with indomethacin (Brooks et al., 1974). Another useful supplement to regular anti-inflammatory therapy is a simple analgesic. Control of pain with regular anti-inflammatory therapy is seldom perfect and a simple analgesic can be used 'on demand', when pains are severe. Suitable drugs for this purpose include aspirin (in analgesic doses) or paracetamol (acetaminophen), or for patients who find aspirin toxic or paracetamol ineffective, the combination of paracetamol and dextropropoxyphene.

The first few weeks or months of treatment of a patient with rheumatoid arthritis are occupied with the search for the ideal symptomatic therapy. Because of the individual variation in response to these drugs, it is often necessary to try a number of different compounds before finding the most suitable. Each drug should be given for at least 1 week, but those which are ineffective after this time are unlikely to work at all. It is important to assess the efficacy of each change of treatment. If this is not done, the patient simply accumulates treatments and it is impossible to decide which, if any, is having an effect.

2. Persistently Active or Progressive Disease

The next decision to be taken is whether to use penicillamine or gold or one of the similar specific 'long-term' compounds (chapter III). This decision should be taken after about 6 months of disease. Before this time, the course of the disease is unpredictable and spontaneous remissions may occur. Once the disease has been present continuously for 6 months, it is likely to remain. The indications for this type of treatment are given in table I.

Patients with persistently uncontrolled disease, despite the use of a wide range of non-steroidal anti-inflammatory analgesics, represent a common indication. Such patients have severe pain but there should also be evidence of active inflammation of joints with prolonged morning stiffness, fatigue, swollen warm joints with effusions and synovial proliferation, anaemia and a raised ESR. Patients with early rheumatoid arthritis should be kept under close observation to detect the earliest signs of progressive disease. Once fixed deformities have developed or cartilage has been destroyed, the changes are irreversible and the amount of improvement to be expected is limited.

The earliest sign of developing deformities should represent an urgent indication for this type of drug therapy — this may be the appearance of ulnar drift of the

Table I. Indications for long-term treatment of rheumatoid arthritis with penicillamine, gold or similar compounds

1. Persistently uncontrolled disease despite adequate anti-inflammatory therapy.
2. Progressive disease.
   a) Developing deformities or permanent joint changes.
   b) Deteriorating X-rays.
3. Excessive steroid requirements.
4. Troublesome extra-articular features.

fingers, flexion deformities of the knees or deformities of any other joint. Clinical evidence of irreversible anatomical changes in joints is particularly difficult to assess, and severe changes may take place without dramatic external manifestations. The development of restriction of movement in any joint usually indicates progressive changes but X-rays are perhaps the best guide. X-rays of the hands, wrists and feet should be assessed before and after 6 months treatment, with X-rays of other joints if there is a clinical suspicion of progressive changes. Patients who show evidence of radiological deterioration with the development of new erosions or loss of joint space should on present evidence receive penicillamine.

Two minor indications for specific treatment with 'long-term' agents are excessive corticosteroid requirements and troublesome extra-articular disease. Penicillamine, gold and related drugs have a potent steroid-sparing effect and are a useful aid to the reduction of corticosteroid dosage in patients who are receiving large doses. They are also useful for troublesome nodules, synovitis around joints, ligaments, tendons and bursae, lymphadenopathy, peripheral neuropathy and sometimes other extra-articular features.

A common problem is the patient with long-standing disease who still has severe pain. Drugs like penicillamine may be very useful, even in the presence of permanent anatomical changes if there is also active synovitis. Removal of the active disease in such patients may relieve pain as well as morning stiffness and local inflammatory features. As in patients with early disease, an assessment must be made of the relative components of active inflammation and anatomical change in the production of symptoms.

Response to drugs like penicillamine and gold is unpredictable. About 80% of patients respond but this is not determined by age, sex, duration of disease or by serological status. It is best to regard such treatment as a therapeutic trial and it is always necessary to review the results of such treatment after about 6 months. For this reason, careful documentation of disease severity before treatment is essential since patients often forget how bad they were before treatment — they are reminded only when the disease returns after treatment has been stopped.

The first choice of drugs from this group is, in my opinion, penicillamine. Although it causes more side-effects than gold, it can more often be continued and it has a more pronounced effect on the progression of X-ray changes (Gibson et al., 1976). About 40 % of patients must stop treatment, either because of lack of effect or because of side-effects. Such patients can be treated with gold. There is a strong tendency for patients who fail to respond to penicillamine to fail also with gold and it may be a better plan to use azathioprine in these cases. Penicillamine, gold and azathioprine, in that order, represent at the present time, a suitable therapeutic range for most patients requiring this type of treatment. Occasional patients with severe disease including vasculitis, who fail to respond to these drugs, will need chlorambucil or cyclophosphamide. Some clinicians use other drugs of this type including chloroquine, dapsone and levamisole and further experience with new drugs may alter the order of preference expressed above.

Drugs like penicillamine take several months to exert their effect and during this time it is necessary to continue analgesic and anti-inflammatory drugs. These can safely be continued with penicillamine, gold and immunosuppressive drugs, with one important exception — other drugs which may affect the bone marrow should be avoided, in particular phenylbutazone and oxyphenbutazone. As penicillamine becomes effective, efforts should be made to withdraw the unnecessary symptomatic therapy.

Treatment with all specific 'long-term' drugs like penicillamine requires careful supervision because of their side-effects. A good knowledge of the toxicity of each drug is necessary before treatment is begun (chapter III). For most of these drugs, a monthly blood count is required and urine should be tested for protein at the same time. Because of the side-effects, skilful management is often required to maintain patients on a successful treatment. The aim of such treatment is to suppress the disease process. The disease process uncontrolled lasts, if not for ever, for many years. Treatment with drugs like penicillamine must therefore be continued either for ever or at least for many years.

3. Role of Corticosteroids

Systemic corticosteroids have little place in the management of rheumatoid arthritis. In doses required to suppress the disease, Cushing's syndrome is inevitable (see chapter IV). Added to this, corticosteroids do not improve the eventual outcome and without such a benefit, the risks are not justifiable. The rheumatoid patient has enough problems without adding hypertension, weight gain, skin changes, osteoporosis, diabetes mellitus, cataracts and mental disturbances. The short course of steroids must also be condemned. Many short courses of a modest dose of corticosteroids have turned into a lifetime of treatment because it is so difficult to withdraw therapy.

Local corticosteroid injections are useful in rheumatoid arthritis and are discussed in chapter V.

It is occasionally useful to give 5mg of prednisolone at night as an alternative to indomethacin for relief of night pain and morning stiffness. Very occasionally, and particularly in the explosive type of rheumatoid arthritis which occurs in the elderly, a very small dose of prednisolone (2.5mg 3 times daily) is dramatically effective. If either of these regimens is used, the patients' response should be assessed after 1 week of treatment. If it has not proved very effective, it should be stopped immediately; if it is continued, patients should be warned of the danger of increasing the dose, which must be kept at the lowest possible level. There is a heavy burden of responsibility on the clinician who starts a patient with rheumatoid arthritis on systemic corticosteroids.

4. Role of Other Types of Drug

Some other drugs are required as supportive measures in rheumatoid arthritis (chapter XXI). Benzodiazepines such as diazepam are a useful addition to night-time treatment with indomethacin or analgesics to improve sleep. It must be stressed however, that provision of pain relief is the first essential for patients in whom pain is the cause of loss of sleep. Oral iron is sometimes needed for anaemia, although large quantities of iron are wasted on the unsuspecting rheumatoid population, whose anaemia is more often related to the activity of their disease. Evidence of iron deficiency must therefore be obtained before iron is used. Intravenous iron should rarely or never be used since it may exacerbate arthritis. Antidepressants are sometimes useful for the more than usually depressed rheumatoid.

5. The Late Stages of the Disease

In the later stages of the disease, the treatment priorities change. Symptoms no longer arise only from active inflammation of joints but also from mechanical problems, the result of anatomical and structural damage to the joint. It is important to try to assess the relative component of these 2 factors in the symptoms. Patients with active inflammatory disease have prominent stiffness, signs of inflammation of joints and a raised ESR. Those with mechanical problems have pain which is abolished by rest and brought on by particular activities.

The important observation that aspirin was more effective than pethidine (meperidine) [Fremont Smith and Bayles, 1965] applies to early disease. In the late stages, a potent anti-inflammatory effect is less important and analgesics may be just as effective as anti-inflammatory drugs. Drugs like penicillamine are obviously not effective in patients whose symptoms result from mechanical problems. In such patients, the less toxic anti-inflammatory drugs such as propionic acid derivatives are preferred but simple analgesics are often very effective. Occasionally, an oral narcotic drug is required in a patient with very severe disease. It is in this stage of the disease that surgery is important and when all possible resources must be brought to bear on a disabled patient to maintain his way of life as normal as possible.

6. Conclusions

An aggressive approach to the treatment of rheumatoid arthritis is much more appropriate today than it was even 10 years ago. There are many more drugs available so that many more patients should be able to find a drug which suits them. There are drugs like penicillamine which are capable of altering the course of the disease in some patients and these must not be withheld if there is evidence of progression. If these drugs were less toxic, one would surely advocate their use as the first line treatment of the disease, when the capacity for improvement is greatest. It is never justified to wait for permanent changes and a patient who shows unfavourable prognostic signs should be treated at the earliest possible time.

Patients with rheumatoid arthritis take many pills. Their therapeutic regimen should be reviewed regularly to ensure that all drugs taken are really needed, and that they are given in the lowest possible maintenance dose.

References and Recommended Reading

Anon.: Is all aspirin alike? Medical Letter 16: 57 (1974).

Brooks, P.M.; Bell, M.A.; Sturrock, R.D.; Famaey, J.P. and Dick, W.C.: The clinical significance of indomethacin-probenecid interaction. British Journal of Clinical Pharmacology 1: 287 (1974).

Fremont-Smith, K. and Bayles, T.B.: Salicylate therapy in rheumatoid arthritis. Journal of the American Medical Association 192: 1133 (1965).

Gibson, T.J.; Huskisson, E.C.; Wojtulewski, J.A.; Scott, P.J.; Balme, H.W.; Burry, H.C.; Grahame, R. and Hart, F.D.: Evidence that D-penicillamine alters the course of rheumatoid arthritis. Rheumatology and Rehabilitation 15: 211 (1976).

Huskisson, E.C.: Reports on Rheumatoid Diseases, No. 54 (Arthritis and Rheumatism Council, London 1974).

Huskisson, E.C.: in Inflammatory Arthropathies (Excerpta Medica, Amsterdam 1976).

Huskisson, E.C.: Wojtulewski, J.A.; Berry, H.; Scott, Jane; Hart, D.F. and Balme, H.W.: Treatment of rheumatoid arthritis with fenoprofen: Comparison with aspirin. British Medical Journal 1: 176 (1974).

Huskisson, E.C.; Woolf, D.L.; Balme, H.W.; Scott, Jane and Franklyn, Sue: Four new anti-inflammatory drugs: responses and variations: British Medical Journal 1: 1048 (1976).

Chapter IX

Osteoarthrosis

Drug treatment is very inadequate in osteoarthrosis. There are no drugs which have any effect on the outcome of the disease, as penicillamine appears to have in rheumatoid arthritis. Nevertheless, drugs are, in most cases, the major weapon which clinicians use to relieve the symptoms of this disease. Surgery is also used but is limited to certain joints such as the hip and to late cases with severe disability. Even if every osteoarthritic joint could be replaced, there would still be many drugs required by patients awaiting their operations. Apart from drugs and surgery, there are physical measures, such as heat, cold, exercises, hydrotherapy and physical aids, such as walking sticks, which also play a part in the total treatment of the osteoarthritic patient.

Osteoarthrosis is a very common condition. It affects about 50 % of the population if X-ray changes are considered and about half of all patients with X-ray changes have symptoms (Kellgren and Lawrence, 1958). It is the major cause of disability resulting from locomotor disease (Thompson et al., 1974) and is a major cause of loss of time from work and of patients seeing doctors and requiring drugs.

It is important to remember that osteoarthrosis is not a well defined disease but a disease process with multiple causes — to emphasise this concept, it has been called 'joint failure'. Thus, a variety of disease processes may lead to cartilage deterioration, including congenital anatomical abnormalities, diseases of childhood such as Perthes' disease, traumatic and mechanical problems such as fractures through the joint surface, obesity and meniscectomy, crystal deposition in pyrophosphate arthropathy, metabolic abnormalities of cartilage and some other conditions, such as septic arthritis, which damage cartilage (Howell et al., 1976).

1. Analgesics and Pain Relief

The conventional view of osteoarthrosis is of a non-inflammatory condition, associated with ageing, in which 'wear and tear' leads by purely mechanical means to progressive loss of cartilage. The concept of degenerative joint disease emphasises this view and the term 'osteoarthrosis' has been advocated instead of 'osteoarthritis' by purists who see little inflammation in the condition. The effusions were called 'non-inflammatory' and, of course, there was no justification for the use of anti-inflammatory drugs. Some cases are like this. Disease of 1 or 2 joints resulting from a mechanical problem such as a fracture, and particularly the late stage of osteoarthrosis, like the late stage of rheumatoid and other arthropathies, is often a purely mechanical problem. In this stage of the disease, patients have pain which is clearly related to activities of various types and they do not have stiffness in the morning or after sitting. Effusions are not usually present in the joints and there are no other signs of inflammation. In this stage of the disease, analgesics are certainly the treatment of choice. They are also suitable for patients with pain which is mild or intermittent. A patient with pain which is produced by certain activities will probably be best treated with a simple analgesic to be taken on demand.

The choice of simple analgesics has been discussed in chapter VI. As with all analgesics and anti-inflammatory drugs, there is a wide individual variation in response and the object of the selection process is to find the right drug for each individual patient. Paracetamol (acetaminophen) is widely used for this purpose and represents a well-tolerated mild analgesic which is safe in therapeutic doses. The dose required is 1g repeated every 4 to 6 hours when necessary. Aspirin in a dose of 600mg is slightly more effective and probably not quite so well tolerated. Much has been written about the poor tolerance of aspirin but this usually refers to its use in anti-inflammatory doses. Doses of 2.4g daily or less are probably well-tolerated by most patients, who rely on aspirin or an aspirin-containing combination as their household analgesic.

For patients in whom paracetamol is not sufficient, and who cannot tolerate aspirin, the combination of paracetamol (325mg) and dextropropoxyphene (32.5mg) is useful (Huskisson, 1974). It is as effective as aspirin and well-tolerated at therapeutic dosage. Aspirin-containing combinations have no obvious advantages over aspirin alone, although many patients have their own particular favourite. Floctafenine is a recently introduced analgesic with comparable effectiveness to aspirin (Huskisson and Scott, 1977). One can also use non-steroidal, anti-inflammatory analgesics like naproxen or fenoprofen which have good analgesic activity and can be taken in single doses on demand (Wojtulewski et al., 1975). Narcotic drugs should in general be avoided because of their addictive potential, but perhaps clinicians have become over cautious! For an elderly patient who is not amenable to surgery, life may be transformed by the use of an oral narcotic agent such as the combination of dipipanone and cyclizine and in patients with severe disease, the effects of non-narcotic analgesics are sometimes very disappointing.

2. Inflammation and Anti-inflammatory Drugs

In many cases of osteoarthrosis there is an obvious inflammatory component. This has often been regarded as an uncommon variant of the condition which has been described as 'primary generalised osteoarthritis' (Kellgren and Moore, 1952) and as 'inflammatory osteoarthritis' (Ehrlich, 1975). In fact, it is very common to find some evidence of inflammation. Many patients have stiffness in the morning or after sitting, effusions, or in the early stages of the disease, 'hot Heberden's nodes'. The latter are red swollen tender distal interphalangeal joints; they remain inflamed for months or years, leaving 'knobbly' fingers when the inflammation passes. Further, osteoarthrosis often responds to anti-inflammatory drugs like indomethacin, which may be much more effective than simple analgesics. Thus, the non-steroidal, anti-inflammatory analgesics provide very useful therapy for many cases of osteoarthrosis. This is especially true in the early stages of the disease when inflammation is most marked.

The usual principles apply to the selection of anti-inflammatory drugs for osteoarthrosis. The principle of using the safest and best-tolerated drugs first is particularly attractive in this disease. The more potent but more toxic anti-inflammatory agents are not required. Propionic acid derivatives like naproxen, fenoprofen, ibuprofen or ketoprofen are therefore ideal. Perhaps their anti-inflammatory activity is less than that of phenylbutazone or aspirin but they provide good pain relief at an acceptable level of side-effects. It is necessary to find the right drug for each individual patient and one must therefore sometimes try several drugs before finding the most suitable. Other drugs with properties similar to the propionic acid derivatives and in particular a low incidence of side-effects, are equally reliable. These include tolmetin, azopropazone and sulindac (see further chapter II).

When night pain is prominent, and occasionally for morning stiffness, indomethacin can be given in a large dose at night. Other non-steroidal anti-inflammatory drugs can also be used for this purpose, including in particular ketoprofen. These can be combined with a hypnotic such as diazepam, flurazepam or nitrazepam to improve sleep. Intra-articular therapy (chapter V) plays a much smaller part in osteoarthrosis than in rheumatoid arthritis and there is no good evidence that corticosteroids are effective. Nevertheless, in a patient with a knee effusion, aspiration and injection of a suitable corticosteroid preparation often seems to be useful.

Rapid radiological deterioration of osteoarthritic hips has been described in patients receiving anti-inflammatory drugs, particularly indomethacin. Such rapid deterioration may also occur in patients not receiving anti-inflammatory drugs and the existence of this so-called analgesic arthropathy remains unproved. Certainly, there is no merit in withholding effective therapy from patients in pain.

3. Conclusion

Drug therapy is the most logical first step in patients with generalised osteoarthrosis and an anti-inflammatory drug like a propionic acid derivative is the most logical first choice. When the disease is localised to 1 or 2 joints, physical measures may be more suitable and the use of walking aids, weight reduction and exercises must always be considered. Surgery may be required in the later stages of the disease and at this stage, anti-inflammatory agents tend to be less successful and simple analgesics are often the mainstay of pain relief.

References and Recommended Reading

Ehrlich, G.E.: Osteoarthrosis beginning with inflammation. Definitions and correlations. Journal of the American Medical Association 232: 157 (1975).

Howell, D.S.; Sapolsky, A.I.; Pita, J.C. and Woessner, J.F.: Pathogenesis of osteoarthritis. Seminars in Arthritis and Rheumatism 5: 365 (1976).

Huskisson, E.C.: Simple analgesics for arthritis. British Medical Journal 4: 196 (1974).

Huskisson, E.C. and Scott, P.J.: Floctafenine: A new analgesic for use in rheumatic diseases. Rheumatology and Rehabilitation 16: 54 (1977).

Kellgren, J.H. and Lawrence, J.S.: Osteoarthrosis and disk degeneration in an urban population. Annals of the Rheumatic Diseases 17: 388 (1958).

Kellgren, J.H. and Moore, R. Generalised osteoarthritis and heberden's nodes. British Medical Journal 1: 181 (1952).

Thompson, M.; Anderson, M. and Wood, H.N.: Proceedings: Locomotor disability — a study of need in an urban community. British Journal of preventive and Social Medicine 28: 70 (1974).

Wojtulewski, J.A.; Hart, F.D. and Huskisson, E.C.: Fenoprofen in treatment of osteoarthrosis of hip and knee. British Medical Journal 2: 475 (1974).

Chapter X

Gout

In gout, there is an abnormality in urate metabolism which results in high and sustained serum urate levels. In some cases of primary gout there is evidence of overproduction, in some of under-excretion and in some both overproduction and under-excretion. Precipitation of urate crystals into joints, renal tubules and tissues may result in acute arthritis, renal (uric acid) calculi and tophi. Renal calculi occur in a minority of patients and may actually precede the acute attack, whereas tophi are usually late manifestations of gout occurring some years after the initial acute arthritis and affecting today about 20% of untreated patients. Treatment of gout falls under three main headings: (a) treatment of the acute attack, (b) prevention of acute episodes, and (c) dissolution of tophaceous deposits.

1. Treatment of Acute Attack

Acute gout is an inflammatory reaction of the tissues due to deposition of crystals of monosodium urate. In most cases it is a primary disease, less often it is secondary to polycythaemia, myeloid metaplasia and rarely chronic granulocytic leukaemia.

1.1 General Prinicples of Treatment

Whatever the type of gout, primary or secondary, whether in low urate excretors or high urate producers, the treatment of the acute episode is the same — the use of an effective well tolerated anti-inflammatory agent in full dosage early in the attack at the very first sign of acute gout. Allopurinol and uricosuric agents should be continued as usual if the patient is already being so treated, but they should not be started during an acute attack, which they may exacerbate. Aspirin has no place in the acute attack. Low doses do not ease symptoms and increase urate levels in the serum, and high doses (around 5g daily), although producing uricosuria do not ease symptoms and may aggravate them.

The most effective agents are phenylbutazone or oxyphenbutazone, indomethacin and the corticosteroids, and more recently naproxen has proven its worth. Ketoprofen, sulindac and other non-steroid anti-inflammatory agents have also proven effective in some cases. Whatever agent is used, it should be started as early as possible in the attack. For this reason, like the diabetic's insulin and the anginal patient's glyceryl trinitrate, the anti-inflammatory agent should be always in the patient's pocket or hand baggage wherever he goes, for all too often gout strikes when the patient is far from home and at a time when pharmacies are closed.

1.2 Routine Investigations

Every gouty patient should have his renal function assessed in the process of discovering what type of primary gout he has and how effective renal clearance of urate is in his case. In addition, it is a wise plan, *between attacks,* to take 2 or 3 test doses of the anti-inflammatory drug selected for future attacks to assess his reaction to it. Patient tolerance of indomethacin and colchicine, for instance, varies considerably. Saturday night and Sunday morning are suitable times for this test as occasional patients react to the large doses of indomethacin; for instance, with headaches and unpleasant cerebral sensations which may even interfere with automobile driving. Gastrointestinal and other reactions may occur with this and other agents.

1.3 The Drugs Available

1.3.1 Indomethacin

If test dosing has proved satisfactory, at the first sign of an acute attack, 50mg of indomethacin with food should be taken; followed thereafter by 25 to 50mg after each meal 3 or 4 times a day, depending on tolerance and therapeutic effect, with 75 to 100mg on retiring by mouth or suppository. Higher doses may be needed in some cases and 100mg 4 to 6-hourly are advocated by some on the grounds that initial high doses are more effective in rapidly controlling symptoms and in acute gout are better tolerated than in other conditions.

In each case, a patient's tolerance has to be assessed by his response during his first few attacks, for individual response both as regards efficacy and tolerance are very variable. Impaired renal clearance of the drug will increase side-effects (chapter II; sect. 4.2). As the attack comes under control, indomethacin is gradually withdrawn, but if minor symptoms persist, it should be continued for several days at lower dosage, such as 25mg 2 or 3 times a day. It is wise to continue such low dosage for 48 hours after all symptoms have subsided. Patients intolerant of indomethacin by mouth but tolerant by rectum, may be given a 100mg suppository morning and evening. Side-effects are less common at night by this route as the patient falls asleep, but may occur more readily in the day. In such cases, half a suppository may be administered 2 to 3 times in the day.

1.3.2 Phenylbutazone and Oxyphenbutazone

The initial daily divided dose of 600mg by mouth of either drug may be raised to 800mg in resistant cases or patients of large body size, and the first dose of 200mg may be increased to 300mg or even 400mg to produce a more rapid effect in such patients. Dosage is then reduced on day 2 to 500mg daily, and subsequently reduced by 100mg daily, although it is wise to continue for at least 48 hours at a low dosage, such as 100mg twice daily, after symptoms have completely subsided. If slight but true gouty symptoms persist, dosage may be continued at 100mg twice or thrice daily until they subside, but the clinician should be sure that they are gouty and not due to chronic osteoarthrosis of the affected joint.

Prolonged treatment with these drugs carries a risk of serious haematological hazards which are exceptionally rare with short periods of therapy given only occasionally. Both phenylbutazone and oxyphenbutazone should be given with or after food, but suppositories (250mg) of both substances are available, as are preparations of phenylbutazone for intramuscular injection. Such injections are often very effective and treatment may be initiated in this way.

1.3.3 Colchicine

Although colchicine had been in use for centuries without effective rivals in the treatment of acute gout, it was superseded as first choice when phenylbutazone and then indomethacin became available. Many patients suffer gastrointestinal upset before effective relief is obtained, and diarrhoea usually tends to be annoying and occasionally incapacitating. The dosage which produces relief also frequently causes considerable diarrhoea. Boardman and Hart (1965) therefore ranked colchicine third after indomethacin and phenylbutazone. Nevertheless, some patients do well on colchicine and prefer it. In acute episodes, 1mg may be given immediately by mouth, followed in 1 to 2 hours by a further 1mg; thereafter 0.5mg every 1 to 2 hours for a further 3 doses, then 0.5mg every 2 to 3 hours until relief is obtained or 6mg (12 tablets) have been taken or the patient has diarrhoea.

Again, there is considerable individual variability in response to the drug and treatment programmes have to be individualised in regard to tolerance and effectiveness. Its tendency to cause severe diarrhoea limits its use more than any other factor. Colchicine is degraded by exposure to light and only stable, properly stored preparations will be effective.

1.3.4 Naproxen, Ketoprofen and Sulindac

It has recently been shown that naproxen is an effective agent in acute gout (Sturge et al., 1977). It may be given by mouth in a dose of 750mg (3 tablets) immediately, then 250mg 8-hourly with food; the drug being gradually withdrawn as symptoms come under control. Other non-steroidal anti-inflammatory agents such as ketoprofen (Doury et al., 1975) and sulindac (Diamond et al., 1977), have also been used with good effect.

1.3.5 Corticosteroids and Corticotrophin

In a few cases none of the non-steroidal anti-inflammatory agents prove adequate and in such cases corticosteroids (or corticotrophin) may be used. Because of their hormonal side-effects, it is best to reserve these agents for such resistant cases, which may otherwise run on to a persistent subacute or chronic inflammatory condition, very painful and incapacitating. Such cases may persist for several weeks or months. Although rare today, they were not uncommon 20 years and more ago.

If corticotrophin is used, an initial intramuscular injection of 0.5mg of the synthetic preparation tetracosactrin may be given, or in very resistant cases 0.75 to 1mg; dosage being reduced to 0.3 to 0.5mg daily, then 0.2mg and 0.1mg when symptoms are slight, intramuscular injection being discontinued after symptoms have been fully controlled for 3 days. Rebound attacks occur more readily after discontinuing corticosteroids than after non-corticosteroid therapy. Use of ACTH involves a similar programme of intramuscular injections, starting around 60 to 80 international units, reducing by 10 units daily.

If oral prednisolone is used to control such resistant attacks of gout, it may be necessary to start with 50 to 60mg daily in divided dosage, reducing by 10mg then 5mg daily, raising dosage slightly if symptoms exacerbate, and continuing at minimal dosage of 5mg daily for 3 days after symptoms have completely subsided. Other oral corticosteroids in equivalent dosage may be used instead of prednisolone (chapter IV).

It must be re-emphasised that corticosteroid therapy should only be tried if other agents have failed and the inflammatory condition is truly active gout and not an acute infective condition which may closely resemble gout or be superimposed on it. In such cases, appropriate antibiotics will be necessary, and possibly surgery. Corticosteroid therapy is today very rarely necessary, the non-steroid anti-inflammatory agents providing satisfactory control of attacks in almost all cases.

2. Prevention of Acute Episodes

While the ultimate prevention of acute attacks of gout depends upon the restoration of a normal serum urate concentration, other agents, which may have no effect upon urate metabolism, may reduce the tendency to the recurrence of acute attacks.

2.1 Prophylaxis of Recurrent Attacks

Of these agents, low-dose colchicine may be useful over an extended period. Occasionally, there is a place for the use of indomethacin or phenylbutazone between acute attacks.

2.1.1 Colchicine

The daily administration of a sub-toxic dose of colchicine (usually 0.5mg twice daily) will reduce the frequency of acute attacks of gout (Yu and Gutman, 1961). This applies both in subjects who are hyperuricaemic and in subjects whose serum urate has been restored to within the normal range by treatment. Thus, the use of prophylactic colchicine is a useful addition to all other forms of treatment, both prior to the introduction of urate normalising therapy (section 3) and during the first year or two of its administration. My policy is to continue it for at least 12 months after the last acute attack of joint pain.

2.1.2 Indomethacin

Just as indomethacin is useful in treating acute attacks of gout, it can also be used for recurrent acute attacks which may occur prior to or following the introduction of urate normalising therapy. Depending upon the degree of joint inflammation, the dose of indomethacin may need to be close to that used for an acute attack of gout (section 1.3.1) and therapy may need to be continued at a lower dose level for a longer period than would have been used when the acute attacks were followed by a complete remission. However, by and large, indomethacin should not be needed on a regular long-term basis in subjects with gouty arthritis once the hyperuricaemia has been corrected for some months; unless there are additional complicating factors such as chronic gout or superimposed osteoarthrosis.

2.1.3 Phenylbutazone

Although phenylbutazone in high dosage is both anti-inflammatory and uricosuric in acute gout, such doses (600 to 800mg/day) are associated with an unacceptably high incidence of side-effects if continued for a long period. A similar attitude to prolonged therapy with moderate doses of phenylbutazone (200 to 300mg/day) might be followed in chronic gout as has been applied above to indomethacin, except that indomethacin has less potential for haematological complications.

2.2 Restoration of a Normal Serum Urate Concentration

It is uncommon for acute attacks of gout to recur after the serum urate has been restored to within the normal range (preferably of the order of 0.35mmol/L or 6mg/100ml or less) for 12 months or more. Drug therapy to achieve a normal serum urate concentration (section 3.2) has now been available for many years, but there are still many patients with recurrent gouty arthritis whose serum urate has not been controlled satisfactorily. Thus, the problem is not merely the availability of effective drugs and it appears there may not be an adequate appreciation of the rationale behind this form of treatment. The following aspects are set out to enable a more rational approach towards the prevention of chronic gout.

1) *The administration of drugs to normalise the serum urate concentration is a life-long commitment to regular therapy.* Hence, considerable thought must be given by a clinician before instituting such a regimen. Such a prolonged course of therapy also demands both an assessment of the causative factors in the individual patient, as well as education of the patient in understanding his disease.

2) *To undertake a course of daily therapy for the rest of his life, a patient must be completely convinced of its necessity.* He must realise that withdrawal of treatment will cause a return of his hyperuricaemia which is likely to be followed by a recurrence of acute gout.

3) *Both the clinician and the patient should carefully assess the risks which might occur without treatment.* These can be assessed as follows (Emmerson, 1975):

a) *Recurrent gouty arthritis:* This is not life-endangering but may be very troublesome and incapacitating. It is easier for the patient to appreciate this risk after he has had more than 1 attack. The risk increases with increasing degrees of hyperuricaemia.
b) *Renal calculus disease:* Patients with gout have an increased risk of developing renal calculi. In some cases, the calculus may precede the first acute attack of gout. The development of a renal calculus could persuade both clinician and patient to introduce treatment sooner than would otherwise occur. However, the risk of developing renal colic is not so great as to modify treatment in a person who has never been so affected.
c) *Renal disease and hypertension:* While up to 50% of patients with gouty arthritis have hypertension and up to 25% have evidence of renal disease, the risk of developing these complications in an untreated individual with gout with normal renal function is difficult to assess. These complications seem to be a particular hazard in young overproducers or in subjects with a poor urine volume, and occur with increased frequency in those who have recurrent acute attacks or who have developed tophi. With careful observation of the degree of hyperuricaemia, the development of these complications is unlikely within the first few years of recurrent acute attacks of gout. Patients with serum urate concentrations persistently over 0.6mmol/L may be particularly at risk (Emmerson, 1976).
d) *Vascular disease:* Gout being a syndrome due to a heterogeneous variety of conditions, the risk of vascular disease in gouty subjects is also difficult to quantitate. On evidence currently available, it seems that both hypertension and hyperlipidaemia are more important risk factors in the development of vascular disease than hyperuricaemia. The presence of either of these other 2 factors would thus demand priority in management over hyperuricaemia. When they have been controlled, the hyperuricaemia may have become of less significance.

2.3 Correctable Factors in Hyperuricaemia

As the commencement of treatment with urate-lowering drugs is a commitment to between 20 and 40 years of daily therapy, there is good justification for assessing aetiological factors in a patient's hyperuricaemia and correcting them where possible. In the assessment of the causes of a patient's hyperuricaemia, the following factors need to be considered:

2.3.1 Drugs

Therapy with thiazides promotes hyperuricaemia which may be sufficient to elevate the serum urate from a value which will not cause gouty arthritis to one which will (Steele and Oppenheimer, 1969; Manuel and Steele, 1974). Thus, in a patient with hypertension, the antihypertensive therapy may need to be reviewed and a decision made concerning whether the drug treatment is optimum. It may not always be either necessary or desirable to stop thiazide therapy; on other occasions, however, it may be as simple to control the hypertension with other drugs, such as β-adrenoceptor blocking drugs, which do not promote such hyperuricaemia. If the decision is made to continue therapy with drugs which aggravate hyperuricaemia, the management of the patient will be exactly the same as if the decision had been made to stop these drugs although restoration of a normal serum urate concentration will be made more difficult. Similar considerations apply to the associated use of other drugs such as low dose aspirin or phenylbutazone therapy (see chapter VII; sect. 2.3).

2.3.2 Poor Urine Volume

Urate excretion falls when the urine flow rate is less than 1ml/min. Many normal subjects excrete urine at a lower rate than this, even during waking hours and many more have urine flow rates of less than this during sleep. Thus, the habit of maintaining a large urine flow rate should be acquired early by any person who has had attacks of gout.

2.3.3 Obesity

Obesity is associated with an increase in urate production and usually a decrease in renal excretion of urate (Emmerson, 1973); both of these factors may be corrected by weight loss. Weight loss may also be associated with a reduced need for antihypertensive therapy. The appreciation of the need for weight loss demands a review of the patient's pattern of living, including his pattern of eating and his exercise habits. Correction of obesity may also correct any associated hyperlipoproteinaemia which would, in turn, reduce any risk of degenerative vascular disease. Such a modification of ingrained life patterns is a major hurdle for many patients. If it cannot be achieved, there may be no alternative to the earlier introduction of drug treatment for its complications, but this is no substitute for the correction of the cause in those patients who can be so motivated.

2.3.4 Alcohol Consumption

The regular consumption of significant amounts of alcohol on a daily basis promotes hyperuricaemia. This is mainly due to the reduction of renal excretion of urate due to the production of lactate which is an end product of the metabolism of alcohol. However, the purine content of beer may also contribute when consumption becomes large.

2.3.5 Purine Consumption

A purine-free diet is necessary only during investigation. However, common sense suggests that foods with a high purine content should be taken in moderation by any patient who is experiencing any difficulty in the control of hyperuricaemia. In subjects in whom normal concentrations of serum urate can be maintained with ease, diet need not be considered further. However, in searching for the cause of hyperuricaemia, one still finds patients who normally have a high purine intake, some of whom may take a considerable serving of meat 3 times a day. In such patients, it would seem prudent to restrict a meat meal to once daily.

2.3.6 Endocrine Dysfunction

The correction of myxoedema or hyperparathyroidism can sometimes result in the return to normal of an elevated serum urate. The most common syndrome seen in patients with gout in Australia, is associated with obesity, type IV hyperlipoproteinaemia and the regular heavy consumption of beer. When the aetiological role of these various factors in their gout is explained to some individuals, they readily modify these habits, often with dramatic benefit. The majority have no motivation to change their dietary habits, however, and will need to depend upon drugs to maintain normal serum urate concentrations. It is therefore important to look upon the development of an acute attack of gout as something which demands an assessment of the whole health of the individual. The gout itself may be less important than modification of weight and diet in the promotion of health and the prevention of degenerative vascular disease.

3. Practical Management of Recurrent Gouty Arthritis

The considerations enumerated above have been incorporated into the following recommendations for the management of patients with gouty arthritis:

3.1 First Attack of Gout

When the acute attack has subsided completely, the condition itself, its prognosis, and possible aetiological factors are discussed with the patient. Two 24 hour collections of urine are then undertaken after the patient has been on a purine-free diet

Table Ia. Collection of 24-hour urine specimens while on a purine-free diet

1. *Explanatory Notes*
   1) This investigation is important so that the amount of uric acid which your body produces each day can be determined, without any interference from foodstuffs which increase uric acid formation.
   2) The diet is for investigation and is not intended to be permanent.
   3) The two 24-hour collections should be carried out on the last 2 days of a 7 day purine-free diet period. It is usually most convenient to commence the diet on a Monday and collect the urine during the following Saturday and Sunday and to bring the 2 bottles, each containing a complete 24 hour collection, for assay on the Monday. However, any 7 day period will do.

2. *Diet*

   The diet should be selected from the following foods:
   a) Beverages: water, fruit juice, cordials, carbonated drinks (NO tea, coffee, cocoa, beer or alcohol). It is desirable that you maintain a good urine volume throughout the whole period.
   b) Cereals (refined or whole grain) and cereal products: bread, macaroni, spaghetti, arrow-root, sago, tapioca and cakes.
   c) Milk and mild foods: cheese of all kinds.
   d) Sugar and sweets.
   e) Eggs: gelatin.
   f) Butter and fats of all kinds. Polyunsaturated margarine.
   g) Fruits of all kinds.
   h) Vegetables (except all beans, lentils, peas and spinach) lettuce, tomatoes.
   i) Nuts of all kinds — peanut butter.
   j) Vegetable and cream soups — to be made with allowed vegetables and without meat or meat stock.

   The diet thus includes most sugars, starches and fats. Protein is supplied chiefly by eggs and cheese, and partly by bread, fruit and nuts. There is no restriction on the amount of food taken.

3. *None of the Following Foods Should be Taken During the 7 Days of the Diet*
   a) Meats, poultry, fish, sea food.
   b) Sardines, herrings, anchovies.
   c) Liver, kidney, heart, sweetbread, brains.
   d) Meat extract, gravies, vegemite, marmite.
   e) Yeast and beer products, beer, alcohol.
   f) Beans, peas, lentils, spinach, oatmeal.

   After 5 days on the diet, the two urine collections are begun and the diet continued until the collections are completed.

for 5 days as an outpatient and the serum urate and creatinine measured at the end of that time. A copy of the instruction sheets (table Ia and Ib) is given to the patient to facilitate this. These collections permit measurement of the urine volume, the creatinine clearance and the 24 hour urine uric acid excretion. The 2 consecutive specimens enable the reliability of the collections and the results to be assessed. These

Table Ib. How to collect the 24-hour specimens of urine

1. On the day when collection is to begin, empty the bladder completely on arising and note the time. This time will be the commencing time for your collection and, at this time, you should have an empty bladder and an empty collection bottle.
2. All urine passed after this time, up to *and including* the specimen of urine passed at exactly the same time 24 hours later, should be placed into the collecting bottle. This will comprise all the urine which the body has made during that 24-hour peorid. At the end of that collecting time, you should have an empty bladder and a bottle of urine.
3. *You now commence the second 24-hour collecting period.* However, no urine is discarded at the beginning of this collection period, because the last specimen of the previous collection emptied your bladder in preparation for the start of this second 24-hour urine collection. You will again begin the collection time with an empty bladder and the other empty bottle.
4. All urine for the next 24-hour period should be placed into the *second* bottle, up to *and including* the urine at the final completion time 24 hours after the second commencing time. At that stage, you should have an empty bladder and a second bottle containing a 24-hour urine sample.
5. It is important that *all* urine be collected and none be lost. Thus, it is wise to empty the bladder and collect the urine separately before a bowel action.

investigations also enable renal disease to be identified early and steps taken to correct a poor urine volume. At the same time, fasting lipids should be measured and an assessment made of any associated parathyroid or thyroid dysfunction.

The mean 24 hour urine uric acid on a purine-free diet allows a simple classification of patients with gout into those who are producing excessive amounts of urate (the over-producers) and those who have defective renal excretion of urate (the under-excretors) [table II]. Those whose mean 24 hour urine uric acid exceeds 600mg or 3.6mmol per 24 hours are *over-producers* and are probably at particular risk of uric acid crystal formation, both within collecting tubules and within the renal pelvis. Severe over-producers (urine uric acid over 1000mg or 6mmol per 24 hours) are likely to have an abnormality of enzymatic control of purine synthesis. Subjects whose 24 hour urine uric acid is less than 300mg or 1.8mmol per 24 hours can arbitrarily be looked upon as *under-excretors;* those between 300 and 600mg (1.8 and 3.6mmol) per 24 hours are within the normal range and may represent various combinations of over-production and under-excretion (table II).

The value of the measurement of 24 hour urine uric acid excretion is so that over-producers can be recognised early and the risk of renal disease anticipated and prevented. In such patients, allopurinol, rather than uricosuric drugs, is the drug of choice. On the other hand, uricosuric drugs will correct the basic abnormality in those who are primarily under-excretors. In the majority in whom the 24 hour urine urate is within the normal range, a consideration of associated factors (such as hypertension, heavy alcohol consumption etc.) will help indicate which group of drugs is more appropriate, if drugs need to be administered to normalise the serum urate.

Table II. Urinary uric acid excretion on a purine-free diet

Uric acid excretion (mmol/24h)	Type	Cause
>5.5		HGPRTase deficiency Myeloproliferative disorder
3.6-5.4	Over excretor	Overproduction
1.8-3.6	Normal range	Normal production — normal excretion Over production — under excretion Normal production — under excretion
<1.8	Under excretor	Under excretion — inherited or acquired

Following these preliminary investigations, prophylactic colchicine is usually begun and the patient is seen at 3-monthly intervals. At these times, the blood pressure is checked and the progress of any correctable causes assessed. Prior to each visit, an estimation of the serum urate, urea and creatinine is undertaken. The creatinine clearance is measured annually.

3.2 Recurrent Acute Gouty Arthritis

If sufficient hyperuricaemia persists for a sufficient period, further attacks of gout will occur. These will need treatment on their own merits to induce subsidence of the acute attack (section 1). Eventually, these recurrences will persuade the patient that it is necessary to begin regular therapy for the rest of his life with a drug to normalise the serum urate.

3.2.1 Indications for Urate Lowering Drugs

Thus, treatment to restore the serum urate concentration to normal is indicated under any of the following conditions:

1) *When the patient has had sufficient attacks of acute gout that he is convinced that he needs treatment to prevent the attacks,* or

2) *If complications of hyperuricaemia and gout occur.* These could consist of: (a) frequent acute attacks; (b) the development of hypertension; (c) the development of renal insufficiency, or (d) the development of tophi.

The development of any of these complications to a significant degree should be regarded as a failure of treatment and it should be the role of the clinician to control hyperuricaemia and its aetiological factors before such complications develop. Long-term follow-up has shown that these complications are unlikely to occur in patients whose serum urate is consistently less than 0.6mmol/L (10mg/100ml) [Rosenfeld, 1973; Berger and Yu, 1975]. It is therefore safe to watch such patients without urate lowering therapy provided that it is possible to follow the patient regularly and to assess the development of the earliest manifestations of such complications.

3) *In patients with serum urate concentrations persistently greater than 0.6mmol/L (10mg/100ml),* no such evidence that complications are unlikely, is available. In such patients there is an increased risk of acute attacks occurring and of tophus formation and, by analogy, of renal microtophus formation. It is my opinion therefore that persistent hyperuricaemia exceeding 0.6mmol/L (10mg/100ml) in a patient who has suffered acute gout justifies treatment to restore the serum urate to normal.

3.2.2 Choice and Use of Drug

As indicated in section 3.1, it is rational to use allopurinol for over-producers and uricosuric drugs for those whose hyperuricaemia is due primarily to reduced renal excretion of urate. Allopurinol should be used with caution and in lower dosage (chapter VII; sect. 4.2) in patients with renal disease. Uricosuric drugs are contraindicated in patients who are over-producers, in patients who have a poor urine volume or in patients who have ever suffered from renal calculi of any type; they will be ineffective in patients with moderate to considerable degrees of renal insufficiency. Individual tolerance of drugs will also vary, as will the potency of different drugs (fig. 2, chapt. VII), so that it is useful to have a variety of drugs available.

In subjects whose mean 24 hour urine uric acid excretion on a purine-free diet is between 1.8 and 3.6mmol (300 and 600mg) per 24 hours, advice as to the choice of the appropriate drug can be less definite. In the absence of factors which favour one type of drug or contraindicate another, it is my practice to use allopurinol if the mean 24 hour urine urate exceeds 2.7mmol (450mg) per 24 hours and uricosuric agent if the mean urate excretion is less than this value. *However, it is important to note that no therapy should be given to modify the serum urate concentration while any acute joint inflammation is present, because this may perpetuate the joint inflammation.*

This is a simple but well established observation, although the mechanism whereby it occurs is not well understood. When the acute inflammation has subsided completely, drugs to lower the serum urate may then be introduced.

If, after the institution of urate lowering therapy, a patient is persistently troubled by minor joint pains suggestive of gout, one has to choose between either stopping the urate lowering therapy or trying to induce subsidence of the acute gout while continuing this therapy. In the first instance, one would administer indomethacin in a dose calculated to cause subsidence of the acute inflammatory response, and perhaps also reduce the urate lowering drug to a dose which will be causing only a moderate reduction of the serum urate (to approximately 0.36mmol/L or 6mg/100ml). If this is not successful, the drug which is affecting urate concentration must be withdrawn and the patient returned to an asymptomatic state by treatment as for acute gout, before the urate lowering drug is reintroduced in a low dosage.

3.2.3 Monitoring of Therapy

During the first few years of therapy with drugs which normalise the serum urate concentration, it is wise to check the serum urate, urea and creatinine each 3 months, together with the blood pressure. If, during this time the patient has been persistently normouricaemic and normotensive, the interval between visits can be increased. However, the mere prescription of appropriate drugs does not guarantee normalisation of the serum urate and this needs to be checked periodically in each individual to ensure that a normal serum urate is being achieved. Even subjects who have been asymptomatic for 5 years should be reviewed at least annually and the adequacy of treatment in controlling hyperuricaemia confirmed. At such times, patients should also be assessed for the development of any possible complications of the disease or of therapy.

4. Clinical Management of the Acute Crystal Deposition Syndromes

4.1 Calcium Pyrophosphate Dihydrate Crystal Disease

This may present clinically as an acute, subacute or chronic arthropathy, usually of the large joints, especially the knee; calcification of the cartilage of affected joints (chondrocalcinosis) is often seen radiologically (Moskowitz et al., 1973). When it presents as an acute arthritis (sometimes referred to as the pseudo-gout syndrome), it is due to the rupture of subchondrial collections of these crystals, which lead to an inflammatory polymorph response (McCarty et al., 1963). These crystals are identifiable in joint fluid under polarised light as being weakly but positively birefringent (Phelps et al., 1969). More commonly, the symptoms suggest a subacute or chronic arthritis. Calcium pyrophosphate dihydrate crystal disease is found in association with degenerative joint disease, haemochromatosis (Webb et al., 1972), hyperparathyroidism (Pritchard et al., 1977), hypertension, renal disease and urate crystal arthritis. Features of the disease are contrasted with those of sodium urate crystal deposition disease in table III.

Treatment of the acute attack: This usually subsides following complete aspiration of the joint. Sometimes the intra-articular injection of corticosteroids is helpful (see chapter V). Otherwise, non-steroidal anti-inflammatory analgesic drugs such as indomethacin may be used in a dosage similar to that used for acute gouty arthritis (section 1.3.1). Colchicine is occasionally of value, but by no means as predictably as in urate gout.

Table III. Features of crystal-induced arthritis

	Sodium urate crystal deposition disease	Calcium pyrophosphate crystal deposition disease
Crystal	Monosodium urate monohydrate	Calcium pyrophosphate dihydrate
Refringence	Negative, strong	Positive, weak
Syndrome	Acute gout	Pseudo-gout An acute, subacute or *chronic* arthropathy of large joints, especially the knee
Associated diseases	Hyperuricaemia Urate overproduction Urate under-excretion	Degenerative joint disease Haemochromatosis Urate gout Hyperparathyroidism Hypertension Azotaemia
Radiology	Nil or radiolucent area; punched out, juxta-articular erosions	Nil, or chondrocalcinosis articularis (may be asymptomatic)
Pathogenesis	Intra-articular crystal formation, ?precipitation Polymorphs essential	Rupture of subchondral collection of crystals Polymorphs essential
Treatment	Colchicine Indomethacin Phenylbutazone	Arthrocentesis ± Intra-articular steroids Analgesics, especially indomethacin
Prophylaxis	Normalise serum urate	Correct associated disease

Treatment of subacute and chronic arthritis: This is managed with analgesics and measures similar to those used for osteoarthrosis (chapter IX), although the most potent agents such as indomethacin may need to be used for any associated inflammatory episodes.

Prevention lies in determining any causative factors, particularly in identifying the associated diseases mentioned and correcting these factors when possible.

4.2 Calcium Hydroxyapatite Crystal Deposition Disease

The clinical presentation is that of a chronic arthropathy resembling osteoarthrosis upon which acute episodes of inflammatory arthritis, often associated with effusion, may at times be superimposed (Dieppe et al., 1976). The syndrome has been likened to primary generalised osteoarthrosis. Repeated attacks lead to the deposition of radio-opaque material in or around the joints. The crystals of calcium hydroxyapatite are usually too small for identification on light microscopy and are not birefringent in polarised light. They can be identified only by scanning electron microscopy and analysis of the phosphorus to calcium ratio as calculated from energy dispersive microanalysis.

Management is essentially similar to that of other acute crystal deposition syndromes, especially that outlined above for calcium pyrophosphate crystal deposition.

References and Recommended Reading

Berger, L. and Yu, T-F: Renal function in gout. IV. An analysis of 524 gouty subjects including long-term follow-up studies. American Journal of Medicine 59: 605 (1975).

Boardman, P.J. and Hart, F.D.: Indomethacin in the treatment of acute gout. Practitioner 194: 560 (1965).

Diamond, H.S.; Bankhurst, A.D.; Wilkens, R.D.; Godfrey, R.G.; Katz, W.A.; Oliver, J.A.; Shenker, B.M. and Wolfe, F.: Sulindac in the treatment of acute gout. Abstracts XIV International Congress of Rheumatology, p.255 (San Francisco 1977).

Dieppe, P.A.; Huskisson, E.C., Crocker, P. and Willoughby, D.A.: Apatite deposition disease. A new arthropathy. Lancet 1: 266 (1976).

Doury, P.; Pattin, S.; Legros, P. and Guintran, J.L.: Treatment of an attack of gout. Med Armees 3: 139 (1975).

Emmerson, B.T.: Alteration of urate metabolism by weight reduction. Australian and New Zealand Journal of Medicine 3: 410 (1973).

Emmerson, B.T.: Hyperuricaemia — To treat or not. Drugs 9: 141 (1975).

Emmerson, B.T.: Gout, uric acid and renal disease. Medical Journal of Australia 1: 403 (1976).

McCarty Jr., D.J.; Kohn, N.N. and Faires, J.S.: The significance of calcium phosphate crystals in the synovial fluid of arthritic patients: The "pseudo-gout syndrome". I. Clinical aspects. Annals of Internal Medicine 56: 711 (1962).

Manuel, M.A. and Steele, T.H.: Changes in renal urate handling after prolonged thiazide treatment. American Journal of Medicine 57: 741 (1974).

Moskowitz, R.W. and Katz, D.: Chondrocalcinosis and chondrocalsynovitis (pseudogout syndrome). Analysis of twenty-four cases. American Journal of Medicine 43: 322 (1967).

Phelps, P.; Steele, A.D. and McCarty, D.J.: Compensated polarized light microscopy. Journal of the American Medical Association 203: 508 (1968).

Pritchard, M.H. and Jessop, J.D.: Chondrocalcinosis in primary hyperparathyroidism. Annals of the Rheumatic Diseases 36: 146 (1977).

Rosenfeld, J.B.: Effect of long-term allopurinol administration on serial GFR in normotensive and hypertensive hyperuricaemic subjects. Advances in Experimental Medicine and Biology 41B: 581 (1973).

Steele, T.H. and Oppenheimer, S.: Factors affecting urate excretion following diuretic administration in man. American Journal of Medicine 47: 564 (1969).

Sturge, R.A.; Scott, J.T.; Hamilton, E.B.D.; Liyanage, S.P.; Dixon, A. St. J. and Engler, C.: Multicentre trial of naproxen vs. phenylbutazone in acute gout. Abstracts XIV International Congress of Rheumatology, p.94 (San Francisco 1977).

Webb, J.; Corrigan, A.B. and Robinson, R.G.: Haemochromatosis and "pseudogout". Medical Journal of Australia 2: 24 (1972).

Yu, T-F and Gutman, A.B.: Efficacy of colchicine prophylaxis in gout. Prevention of recurrent gouty arthritis over a mean period of five years in 208 gouty subjects. Annals of Internal Medicine 55: 179 (1961).

Further Reading

Emmerson, B.T.: The management of gout. Medical Journal of Australia 1: 475 (1972).

Emmerson, B.T. and Ravenscroft, P.: Abnormal renal urate homeostasis in systemic disorders. Nephron 14: 62 (1975).

Fessel, W.J.: Hyperuricemia in health and disease. Seminars in Arthritis and Rheumatism 1: 275 (1972).

Rastegar, A. and Thier, S.O.: The physiologic approach to hyperuricemia. New England Journal of Medicine 286: 470 (1972).

Spilberg, I.: Current concepts of the mechanism of acute inflammation in gouty arthritis. Arthritis and Rheumatism 18: 129 (1975).

Wyngaarden, J.B.: Metabolic defects of primary hyperuricaemia and gout. American Journal of Medicine 56: 651 (1974).

Chapter XI

Ankylosing Spondylitis and Related Disorders

Although ankylosing spondylitis was at one time considered a variant of rheumatoid arthritis, it is now universally held to be an entirely different type of disorder, with different sex frequency, age groups, tissue typing, different clinical findings, different pathology, different progression and prognosis and, different management. The essence of the disease is its tendency to bony fusion. It is a stiffening disease rather than an erosive one. Since it affects spinal structures and girdle joints rather than intermediate and peripheral ones, it ultimately tends to produce a patient crippled by immobility and fusion of spine, hips and shoulders (Hart, 1975).

It has become apparent in the last 15 years or so that other disorders may assume the spondylitic form: Reiter's disease, psoriatic arthritis, and the arthritis associated with Crohn's disease, ulcerative colitis and Whipple's disease. The subject is well reviewed by Wright et al. (1976). It appears that the ankylosing spondylitic pattern of disease has occurred in the majority of such patients, whatever the associated disease, who have the histocompatibility HLA B27 antigen (Brewerton et al., 1973; Schlosstein et al., 1973). Although the HLA B27 antigen occurs in only around 4 to 7 % of persons in Northern Europe, 88 to 96 % of patients with idiopathic ankylosing spondylitis have this antigen, 76 to 81 % of Reiter's spondylitis, 90 % of psoriatic spondylitis, 72 to 75 % of ulcerative colitic spondylitics, but a lower figure, 27 to 33 % in Crohn's spondylitis. Whipple's disease and Behcet's disease, both associated on occasion with the development of the clinical picture of ankylosing spondylitis, have not been associated with HLA B27 antigen and remain sub judice. But more important is the work of Aho and his colleagues (1973), which demonstrated that in those patients developing spondylitis after yersinial intestinal infection, over 90 % were HLA B27 positive. This strongly suggests that given a patient with certain antigenic tissue predisposition, an infection which is otherwise relatively unimportant may precipitate a chronic rheumatic disorder of the ankylosing spondylitis type.

1. Indications for Drug Treatment

The essential features of the disease which call for medication are:

1) Painful spinal or girdle joint stiffness, aggravated by immobility, particularly at night, and in the early morning.

2) Tenderness on bony pressure over pelvis, ischial tuberosities, sternum and anterior chest wall.

3) Restriction of chest expansion.

4) Painful fasciitis of heels.

5) Pain arising from a hypermobile area between 2 fixed segments of spine.

6) Anterior uveitis.

7) In 1 to 2% of cases cardiac symptoms arising from aortic reflux and conduction defects.

8) Respiratory symptoms.

9) Amyloidosis.

2. Aim of Drug Treatment

The aim of drug treatment in ankylosing spondylitis is to maintain, firstly, full function and, secondly, normal posture. As full a range of spinal and other joint movements as possible should be maintained by an active mobile life and daily exercises, and to enable these to be done, non-steroidal anti-inflammatory analgesics are the most helpful therapeutic agents.

Phenylbutazone and oxyphenbutazone have a prolonged even action and are in the opinion of many sufferers the best drugs to combat the painful stiffness which is the outstanding symptom in this disease. Phenylbutazone in 1952 replaced deep X-ray therapy, which was becoming unpopular at the time due to reports of acute leukaemia arising from its use. However, in turn the pyrazoles came under the same cloud, and, effective drugs though they are for this disease, the risk of aplastic anaemia, thrombocytopenia and leucopenia have made many clinicians seek other agents.

Indomethacin appeared about 1964 and proved effective in ankylosing spondylitis — 25mg after meals 1 to 4 times a day at the lowest effective dose, usually with a loading dose at night of 50 to 100mg with food by mouth or 100mg by suppository. Painful stiffness at night and in the early morning is a major symptom in this disorder and this final dose on retiring is often the most helpful single item in the spondylitic's therapeutic programme. A 1 or 2 nights trial will prove or disprove its efficacy, and the indomethacin nightly suppository has definitely proven its worth in this disorder. Anal irritation occurs in about 1 in 10 cases, but gastric irritation is less likely to occur with suppository than with capsules. Although blood levels are negligible by dawn the relief obtained suggests that the tissue levels of indomethacin are sufficient. The cerebral sensations noted with high dosage are much less common at night as the patient goes into a sounder sleep, simple movements in sleep not waking him as they are rendered less painful or painless.

Alternatives to phenylbuytazone and indomethacin, although usually in the author's experience somewhat less effective, are naproxen, fenoprofen, ketoprofen, ibuprofen, flufenamic acid, alclofenac, sulindac, flurbiprofen and others. In each case a loading dose at night will help the nocturnal and early morning symptoms, for instance with naproxen 250mg in the morning, 500mg on retiring. In general, aspirin in its various forms helps only the milder cases and the simple analgesics ease painful exacerbations only slightly, the anti-inflammatory drugs helping the spondylitic far more.

Whatever drugs are used the aim is to assist in mobilisation of the patient, to enable him to do his work, perform his daily exercises and lead as normal a life as possible. A full active life at work is best for the patient physically, psychologically, socially and financially, and the drug programme of administration is aimed essentially at enabling him to lead such a life.

3. Role of Corticosteroids

Corticosteroids and corticotrophin have little part to play in routine management of this disease but are indicated in certain situations.

1) A nocturnal dose of 5mg prednisolone can be given to control night symptoms if other non-steroidal anti-inflammatory agents prove inadequate.

2) A regular divided daily dose of 7.5mg prednisolone or less, can be used in certain patients not responding to other agents; often those with peripheral joint involvement.

3) Courses of intramuscular corticotrophin or tetracosactrin can be used to control periods of acute exacerbations.

A word of warning is required here. Some of these so-called exacerbations are based on trauma and will, in fact, usually abate spontaneously within 3 weeks. The rigid spine of a spondylitic cannot adapt readily to rapid changes in position and is the more liable to suffer damage, ranging from mild but painful soft tissue lesions to fractures, occasionally fatal. Rarely, the disease may become diffusely and acutely worse and in such cases, if not based on intercurrent infection or mental disturbance, 10 to 14 day courses of corticotrophin or tetracosactrin may be given, preferably in hospital under close medical observation. Dosage varies with the individual case, 40 to 60iu of corticotrophin daily initially, reducing by 5iu daily; or 0.1 to 0.25mg tetracosactrin intramuscularly daily, reducing dosage gradually when acute symptoms are controlled. Only rarely are such courses necessary; the major disadvantage being that the relief obtained may lead to long-term therapy if symptoms do not subside within the 2 week period, with all the attendant hazards of long-term corticosteroid therapy.

4) Local injections of corticosteroid may be useful in certain peripheral manifestations, e.g. painful large effusions into knee joints.

5) Corticosteroids are indicated in the control of anterior uveitis (see below).

4. Treatment of Specific Features of the Disease

The above general drug programme covers basically most of the 8 features of the disease listed above, but a few additional therapeutic points might be made.

The *bony tenderness* over pelvis, chest and elsewhere is usually transient, though often lasting several months. Lytic lesions in bone may underly some of these pains; some are at the enthesis (the muscle and ligamentous insertions), but in others there is no apparent cause for what appears to be a very real bony tenderness, preventing sleep in some cases when the patient turns onto a tender crest of the ilium. Drug treatment is essentially by the non-steroidal anti-inflammatory analgesics listed above. Local deep X-ray therapy in very small dosage, and physical measures, such as a soft cushion under the ischial tuberosities, are of more help. Local injections of analgesics or corticosteroids are seldom helpful or practical.

The *chest restriction* so typical of the disorder is usually not very painful unless there is sustained overbreathing. As this is to be encouraged at all times, so as to diminish the restrictive chest disease which may result, the full programme outlined in section 2 is indicated; drug therapy aiding physical measures and allowing more normal function.

Painful fasciitis is helped more by physical measures, such as soft rubber heels or insoles, or by deep X-ray therapy in very small dosage, than by drugs, although analgesics may play a modest part.

The *hypermobile area* between two fixed segments has to be treated by a period of immobilisation or rest, analgesics as required, but sometimes by surgical fusion. This is one of 4 exceptions to the general therapeutic programme in ankylosing spondylitis of full mobility and activity short of severe strain, the other 3 being trauma, florid exacerbation of the disease and active disease of peripheral joints.

In the treatment of *anterior uveitis,* corticosteroids may be employed locally or systemically. On occasion, the ocular condition may take precedence over all else, but happily, although uveitis is common at some stage of the disease, (25 to 50% in different surveys), it rarely causes permanent impairment of vision.

Aortic reflux may appear suddenly in the course of the disease and be associated with early signs of cardiac failure or it may occur insidiously with less effect on cardiac function. Treatment is with diuretics, digitalis or β-adrenoceptor blocking drugs and other agents according to the case findings.

Respiratory symptoms are usually secondary to the restrictive chest disease caused by the spondylitis or to tuberculosis or other infection, bacterial or fungal. A primary apical fibrosis, said to be part of the disease process, is often symptomless, calling for no therapy other than the basic regimen, outlined in section 2; the only other therapy needed is for any pulmonary infections as they arise. Happily, these are no more common in spondylitic than in the general population.

Amyloidosis is rare and no specific or effective drug therapy for it exists as yet.

5. Treatment of the Secondary Spondarthritides

When patients with psoriatic arthritis, ulcerative colitis, Crohn's disease, Reiter's disease or dysentery develop ankylosing spondylitis, the treatment differs only in its modification in relation to the associated disorder.

5.1 Reiter's Disease

Peripheral joint manifestations are more common, particularly in ankle and knee. The original urethritis and conjunctivitis (if present) will have disappeared and the pattern of disease left behind is ankylosing spondylitis with any or all of the 8 groups of manifestations listed above, but with more peripheral joint involvement which may, for a time at least, interfere with the programme of active mobilisation. The approach to treatment is otherwise identical with that described in section 2.

5.2 Colitic and Crohn's Spondylitis

The management of the spondylitis is modified in this situation by the treatment of the bowel condition; by surgery or drugs. Sulphasalazine and corticosteroids, locally by retention enemata or systemically, are usually needed. The patients are more frail, more anaemic, more likely to be female and are less able to live the active life needed for the treatment of the spondylitis. Nevertheless, a modified programme is usually tolerated. Iron, vitamins and blood transfusions, only rarely needed for the idiopathic or 'primary' spondylitis, are necessary in almost all cases of spondylitis due to ulcerative or Crohn's colitis at some stage. During periods of hospitalisation for surgery, great care must be taken that graded activities and exercises are maintained as far as possible throughout to avoid the increase in stiffening and postural deformities which can develop, sometimes rapidly, during such periods of immobility.

5.3 Psoriatic Arthropathy

This condition differs only in the need for additional treatment of the skin condition and of peripheral joint manifestations, which may be slight in many cases but severe in a few. A few unfortunate patients have all joints of the spine affected as well as the peripheral joints. Here again the full programme may have to be modified in terms of what the patient can do.

6. Conclusion

Gold salts, penicillamine and the antimalarials seem to have no part to play in the treatment of the ankylosing spondylitides, primary or secondary, the antimalarials being contraindicated in psoriatic spondylitis for fear of exacerbating the skin disease. The cytotoxic (immunosuppressive) agents have been used in some severe cases not responding to other forms of treatment, usually of a secondary spondylarthritis, but this is seldom necessary.

Given the active physical programme of full exercise and joint exercises (which, in fact, in most cases is allowing the spondylitic to do what he wants to do) and adequate medication to allow him to function, most spondylitic patients do well. Females usually have more mild disease than males, but the prognosis in both sexes is good, both for life expectation and wage earning, unless there is severe or serious crippling involving hips as well as spine, amyloidosis, cardiac features or serious complications of therapy. It is likely that all the drugs discussed in section 2 and 3 do no more than have a symptomatic effect (improving function and lessening pain and stiffness) and that they leave the basic disease uncured. Depression and anxiety states may occur in patients with ankylosing spondylitis but, although more common in female sufferers than male, are much less common than in patients with rheumatoid arthritis.

References and Recommended Reading

Aho, K.; Ahvonen, P.; Lassus, A.; Sievers, K. and Tillikainen, A.: HL-A antigen 27 and reactive arthritis. Lancet 2: 157 (1973).

Brewerton, D.A.; Hart, F.D.; Nicholls, A.; Caffrey, M.; James, D.C.O. and Sturrock, R.D.: Ankylosing spondylitis and HL-A 27. Lancet 1: 904 (1973).

Hart, F.D.: Inflammatory disease and its control in rheumatic disorders. British Medical Journal 4: 191 (1975).

Schlosstein, L.; Terasaki, P.I.; Bluestone, R. and Pearson, C.M.; High association of an HL-A antigen, W27, with ankylosing spondylitis. New England Journal of Medicine 288: 704 (1973).

Wright, V.; Sturrock, R.D. and Dick, W.C.: Seronegative spondarthritides; in Buchanan and Dick (Eds) Recent Advances in Rheumatology, part 2, p.193 (Churchill Livingstone, Edinburgh 1976).

Chapter XII

Polymyalgia Arteritica

The diseases known as giant cell (cranial) arteritis and polymyalgia rheumatica are, on present evidence, probably 2 phases of the same disorder, an arteritis usually causing arthritic symptoms in girdle joints in the elderly. In some cases, symptoms are patently due to local inflammatory changes in arteries, as in cranial arteritis. In others, the clinical picture is of marked morning stiffness and pain in shoulders and hips, lessening (improving) as the day progresses (polymyalgia rheumatica). In yet others, the picture is a mixed one, but a markedly elevated erythrocyte sedimentation rate occurs in all phases.

In a recent 7 year survey by Myles (1975) in the south of England of 75 cases, the polymyalgic picture was present in 52, cranial arteritis in 5, and a mixed one in 18. This is about the ratio we are seeing of these variants at this time in Great Britain, of what is a not uncommon disease. In the series of Myles there were 7 deaths, all apparently unrelated to the disease or its treatment. This again mirrors what most clinicians find: although polymyalgia arteritica may occlude vital vessels, such as the central artery of the retina or other branches of the ophthalmic artery, a coronary or carotid artery, deaths when they occur are more likely to be due to other unrelated causes than the polymyalgia arteritica. Nevertheless, it is a painful and severely incapacitating disease in the elderly, which usually lasts 1 to 8 years before it spontaneously remits. The risk of blindness, particularly in the cranial arteritic syndrome, is a very real one.

1. Approach to Treatment

Although any effective anti-inflammatory agent will lessen the painful symptoms none are as effective as the corticosteroids and none but corticosteroids at full dosage will prevent occlusion of the central retinal arteries with resultant blindness. For practical purposes, the therapy is, in a word, corticosteroids, in full dosage initially then maintained at the lowest dose which will control the symptoms and normalise the erythrocyte sedimentation rate. It is convenient to have two programmes of therapy.

1) For the straight-forward polymyalgia syndrome — prednisolone 10mg daily in divided dosage, or up to 15mg if necessary initially, dosage being gradually lowered when symptoms are fully controlled and sedimentation rate normalised (0.5 to 1mg reduction every 3 to 4 weeks) or being slightly raised if symptoms return or there are any signs of disease reactivity, slow reduction in dosage being attempted again some weeks later.

2) For cases with cranial symptoms — 20mg initially, or if any visual symptoms are present 40 to 50mg or more daily, reduction in dosage being made when symptoms are fully controlled and sedimentation rate normalised (by 2.5 to 5mg weekly, sometimes more rapidly). The reduction is more gradual when dosage falls below 20mg daily (1mg every 1 to 2 weeks) and when 10mg is reached by 0.5mg every 2 to 4 weeks. These dosage figures are suggestions only and not to be interpreted rigidly, for individual cases vary greatly. Freeman and Russell (1977) suggest a dose of at least 80mg daily for giant cell arteritis as they have seen blindness occur at lower dosage, but this has to be balanced against the risks of high dosage in this age group.

2. Problems in Therapy

The great dangers in therapy are: (1) *in delaying therapy or starting corticosteroid dosage too low,* for blindness may occur in a few days, or even hours, if therapy is delayed, and may also occur if dosage is inadequate i.e. under 30mg prednisolone daily. If cranial or visual symptoms occur at lower dose levels immediate higher dosage is indicated; and (2) *in discontinuing therapy too soon* (Hart, 1975).

Some years ago the natural history of the disease was considered to be 6 to 18 months and therapy was then discontinued. Some cases relapsed immediately, some after a few weeks or months, some flared up in the cranial pattern and a few patients lost their sight. It is wise to maintain a small maintenance dose of 2 to 3mg prednisolone daily, even if sedimentation rates are normal and the patient symptom-free for 3 to 4 years. Alternatively, when there has been no evidence of disease activity for several months, dosage may be gradually phased out down to the last 1mg, on condition that the patient informs his clinician immediately of any return of symptoms. All too often in such cases, symptoms do recur and no immediate action is taken as the clinician is not informed.

Corticosteroids in the elderly have their own very real side-effect risks. Crush vertebral fractures may occur with severe backache, or there may be suppression of the inflammatory features of serious infections, leading to delay in diagnosis. This particularly occurs at higher dose levels of prednisolone over 10mg daily; the risk is still present, though less, at lower dose levels.

The rate of dose reduction must be carefully controlled with the patient's full co-operation. Exacerbation of symptoms, or even more important, the appearance of new visual or cranial ones, must be immediately reported, if necessary by telephone, for sight has been lost in a few hours in some cases.

As patients with polymyalgia arteritica are usually elderly almost all have osteoarthrosis of neck and back and some of the hips. The clinician must therefore always clearly differentiate between the aches and pains of osteoarthrosis and the very different manifestations of polymyalgia arteritica, and although the erythrocyte sedimentation rate is usually of great help many other factors may cause its elevation. Although polymyalgia arteritica is usually a delightful condition to treat, as results are so rapidly apparent within 24 hours and the patient duly grateful, it does carry risks, and there are no specific diagnostic tests, and a very careful follow-up is necessary with full patient co-operation. Arterial biopsies are helpful if positive, but therapy should not be delayed while results are awaited.

References and Recommended Reading

Freeman, A.G. and Russell, R.W.R.: Polymyalgia arteritica. British Medical Journal 1: 1412 (1977).

Hart, F.D.: Visual complications of polymyalgia rheumatica (polymyalgia arteritica). Practitioner 215: 763 (1975).

Myles, A.B.: Polymyalgia rheumatica and giant cell arteritis: A seven year survey. Rheumatology and Rehabilitation 14: 231 (1975).

Wilkinson, I.M.S. and Russell, R.W.R.: Arteries of the head and neck in giant cell arteritis. Archives of Neurology 27: 378 (1972).

Chapter XIII

Systemic Lupus Erythematosus

Systemic lupus erythematosus (SLE) is a syndrome of unknown aetiology and is characterised by inflammation of multiple organ systems: joints, skin, serosa, kidneys and the central nervous system. At least some of the varied organ manifestations appear to result from inflammation of blood vessels. Immune complex mechanisms are involved in the development of lupus glomerulonephritis. The precise nature of antigen antibody complexes that account for hypocomplementaemia and vascular injury is not known, but attention has focussed on autoimmune systems, particularly those involving nuclear antigens (Koffler et al., 1971).

No other disease of man manifests a wider range of autoimmune reactions than does SLE. Immune cytopenias, involving erythrocytes, leukocytes and platelets, are common manifestations and autoimmune specificities for several nuclear and cytoplasmic antigens have been characterised. Antibody reactive with native, double-stranded DNA is the most specific and diagnostic serological feature of SLE. To the extent that the level of anti-DNA antibodies and the degree of hypocomplementaemia correlate with disease activity, these two measurements sometimes influence management decisions (Lightfoot and Hughes, 1976; Schur and Sandson, 1968).

The natural history of SLE has changed enormously over the past few decades. Previously, the syndrome was a hyperacute illness associated with a very high mortality over a period of 1 to 2 years and at necropsy a paucity of anatomical lesions were found. A broadened definition of SLE and the advent of more effective management of acute manifestations are probably responsible for our present concept of the natural history of the disease: it is now a *chronic* disease that affects cardiovascular, renal and central nervous systems. The highest incidence of mortality is associated with chronic glomerulonephritis. Central nervous system disease and sepsis (abetted by modern chemotherapy) are lesser but significant causes of death. There has been a recent appreciation that accelerated and premature atherosclerosis may account for morbidity and mortality in subjects with chronic patterns of disease.

1. Management of Acute Manifestations

1.1 Patients Without Visceral Manifestations

The diagnosis of SLE *per se* does not demand corticosteroid therapy. Patients without visceral manifestations of disease may have rheumatic and constitutional symptoms that can be controlled with non-steroidal anti-inflammatory agents such as aspirin or indomethacin. When aspirin is used to control acute manifestations, there should be an awareness that it may induce hepatotoxicity (Seaman and Plotz, 1976). There is no unanimity regarding the role of antimalarial drugs in the management of SLE, but there is a general impression that chronic cutaneous manifestations are suppressed by drugs such as hydroxychloroquiune, in doses of 200 to 400mg daily. The risk of serious, potentially irreversible, ocular toxicity requires that patients have careful ophthalmological consultations, at least every 6 months during antimalarial therapy (see also chapter III; sect. 4.2).

1.2 Patients with Visceral Manifestations

Corticosteroids are clearly indicated for the management of life-threatening visceral manifestations of SLE: these include glomerulonephritis, central nervous system involvement, vasculitis, severe myositis, and cardiopulmonary disease (table I). Additionally, corticosteroid therapy is the treatment of choice for patients that manifest a toxic febrile state or severe haemolytic anaemia. Attitudes regarding individual preparations of corticosteroids and dosages vary, but when manifestations are acute and severe, prednisolone (or equivalent) in daily doses of 40 to 60mg is the usual recommendation. Regimens that employ either single daily dose or alternate day corticosteroid therapy may be applicable to management of the chronic disease (see section 3), but divided doses (no less than every 8 hours) should be instituted for severe acute disease. When a remission ensues, corticosteroid dosage should be gradually reduced seeking the lowest level that will maintain control of the disease. The effort to diminish dosage should be altered if there are signs of relapse.

The majority of patients with SLE experience remissions. Except in cases of glomerulonephritis and central nervous system disease, long-term, high-dose corticosteroid therapy is therefore not required. The character and management of steroid complications are discussed in chapter IV (sect. 2.3). Of particular importance, is the altered resistance to infection and the uncertainty, in individual patients, in differentiating active SLE from superimposed infection.

The highest levels of morbidity and mortality of SLE are related to renal and central nervous system complications. When organic neurological disease seems unresponsive to corticosteroid therapy (i.e. in the range of 50 to 100mg of prednisolone daily), some have advocated very high doses; as much as several hundred milligrams of prednisolone per day. The case for more moderate therapy of central

Table I. Management of acute SLE

Pattern of disease	Initial therapy	Possible adjuvant therapy
Symptomless with serological abnormalities	Usually no therapy (see text)	—
Mild fever, malaise, rheumatic symptoms	Aspirin (3 to 4g/day) or other non-steroidal anti-inflammatory drugs	Prednisolone (25-50mg/day) if other therapy fails to control disease
High fever, toxic state, and/or serositis, and/or marked haemolytic anaemia	Prednisolone (25-50mg/day)	—
Nephritis — mild and focal glomerulonephritis	Prednisolone (25-50mg/day)	—
Nephritis — severe diffuse glomerulonephritis	Prednisolone (50-100mg/day)	Immunosuppressive drugs (azathioprine or cyclophosphamide; 2 to 3mg/kg/day)
Organic CNS disease	Prednisolone (50-100mg/day)	Consider trial of higher dose prednisolone (200mg/day or immunosuppressive drugs (as above) if disease is unresponsive
CNS dysfunction without neurological signs	Maintain therapy according to other features of disease Observe closely Use psychotherapeutic drugs If other manifestations of active disease are lacking and if CNS dysfunction occurred on corticosteroid therapy, consider gradual reduction of dose	—

nervous system complications of SLE has been summarised (Sergent et al., 1975). The general thesis that the level of therapy should be tailored to the severity and extent of life-compromising disease applies to the management of SLE nephritis. There are indications that nearly all patients with active SLE have renal involvement: the risk of chronic progressive renal failure is highest in patients with diffuse glomerulonephritis. Arbitrary high-dose regimens are not appropriate for patients with mild and focal glomerulonephritis, although such patients should be observed closely for the development of more severe renal involvement.

1.3 Immunosuppressive Therapy

There is no unanimity regarding the indications or the efficacy of drugs such as azathioprine or cyclophosphamide in the management of SLE (Decker et al., 1975; Sztejnbok et al., 1971). Indications for the employment of immunosuppressive agents are based more on clinical impressions than on results of controlled trials. Nevertheless, there are indications that immunosuppressive drugs are suppressive and that their use may permit a lower dose of corticosteroid than would otherwise be required. Toxicity and other aspects of immunosuppressive drugs are discussed in chapter III (sect. 3).

2. Management of Chronic Disease

Since the majority of patients with SLE experience remissions, the regimens and therapy that are appropriate for management of acute manifestations (table I) can usually be modified by gradually seeking a lower dose level of medication over a period of weeks or months. When disease activity is controlled on low to moderate doses of corticosteroids, a trial of single daily dose or alternate day therapy can be tried. If successful, the intermittent regimen can be maintained with subsequent gradual reductions in dose level.

Management of chronic cases involves close observations for signs of active disease, manifest either as clinical or laboratory abnormalities. There are no arbitrary rules that can be applied in the treatment of all patients. As with acute disease, the degree of surveillance and the use of drugs relates to the severity of visceral patterns of disease. If mild rheumatic symptoms develop during the reduction or following cessation of corticosteroid therapy, institution of salicylate treatment is indicated. Because of the high frequency of osteonecrosis in steroid-treated SLE patients, this complication should be considered when there is localised joint pain, especially if it involves a hip or a knee. In some patients, serological abnormalities (hypocomplementaemia and level of antibodies to native DNA) parallel closely clinical signs of disease activity and persistent immunological abnormalities, in an asymptomatic patient, may herald clinical relapse.

The ultimate goal in management of chronic cases is control of all symptoms and laboratory abnormalities with the lowest possible dose level of therapy. Whether or not serological abnormalities alone should alter therapy is a difficult decision that rests with the experience and judgement of the clinician and the pattern of illness that was previously manifest in an individual patient.

References and Recommended Reading

Bulkey, B.H. and Robert, W.C.: The heart in systemic lupus erythematosus and the changes induced in it by corticosteroid therapy. A study of 36 necropsy patients. American Journal of Medicine 58: 243 (1975).

Decker, J.L.; Klippel, J.H.; Plotz, P.H. and Steinberg, A.D.: Cyclophosphamide or azathioprine in lupus glomerulonephritis. A controlled trial: Results at 28 months. Annals of Internal Medicine 83: 606 (1975).

Koffler, D.; Carr, R.I.; Agnello, V.; Thoburn, R. and Kunkel, H.G.: Antibodies to polynucleotides in human sera: antigenic specificity and relation to disease. Journal of Experimental Medicine 134: 294 (1971).

Lightfoot, R.W., Jr. and Hughes, G.R.V.: Significance of persisting serologic abnormalities in SLE. Arthritis and Rheumatism 19: 837 (1976).

Schur, P.H. and Sandson, J.: Immunologic factors and clinical activity in lupus erythematosus. New England Journal of Medicine 278: 533 (1968).

Seaman, W.E. and Plotz, P.H.: Effect of aspirin on liver tests in patients with RA of SLE and in normal volunteers. Arthritis and Rheumatism 19: 155 (1976).

Sergent, J.S.; Lockshin, M.D.; Klempner, M.S. and Lipsky, B.A.: Central nervous system disease in systemic lupus erythematosus. Therapy and prognosis. American Journal of Medicine 58: 644 (1975).

Sztejnbok, M.; Stewart, A.; Diamond, H. and Kaplan, D.: Azathioprine in the treatment of systemic lupus erythematosus. A controlled study. Arthritis and Rheumatism 14: 639 (1971).

Chapter XIV

Vasculitis Syndromes

Vasculitis, to the extent that it is a component of any inflammatory process, is not a disease entity. For the purpose of this discussion, vasculitis syndromes are defined as illnesses in which blood vessel inflammation and necrosis are manifest in multiple organ systems. The clinical syndromes are no more specific than is pneumonitis or nephritis. In many patients, vascular inflammation occurs in a setting of a more complex illness such as rheumatoid arthritis, systemic lupus erythematosus, bacterial endocarditis, drug allergy, paraproteinaemia, etc. (table I). For the most part, vasculitis that is a part of these more complex illnesses is excluded from this discussion; vasculitis associated with rheumatoid arthritis and the syndrome of giant cell arteritis are considered elsewhere (see chapt. VIII, sect. 2; chapt. XII).

The aetiology of diffuse vasculitis syndromes such as polyarteritis nodosa and Wegener's granulomatosis is not known except for the association of HB viral hepatitis infection in approximately one-third of patients with polyarteritis (Sergent et al., 1976). Another possible relationship of vasculitis to a microbial aetiology is suggested by the association of the syndrome with chronic serous otitis media (Sergent and Christian, 1974). Immunological mechanisms seem clearly involved in the pathogenesis of vascular inflammation and injury but, with the exception of drug-induced disease and possibly HBs associated vasculitis, the source and character of the immunogen is not known.

The pattern of organ system involvement in diffuse vasculitis is varied. Any organ may be involved; the central nervous system, peripheral nerves, heart, lungs, kidneys, abdominal viscera, muscles and skin can all manifest ischaemic changes secondary to vasculitis. Many patients with necrotising vasculitis appear to have self-limited courses — a finite period of active disease. If the phase of active disease can be suppressed and if there has not been irreparable damage to vital organs, the prognosis is much better than the literature suggests. The prognosis in general is related to the pattern and severity of organ involvement.

Table I. Vasculitis — Clinical classification

1. *Syndromes characterised by Necrotising Vasculitis*	
'Classic' polyarteritis nodosa	
Wegener's granulomtosis	
Henoch-Schonlein purpura	
Giant cell arteritis	
Aortic arch arteritis	
2. *Syndromes Occasionally Complicated by Necrotising Vasculitis*	
Rheumatic diseases	Hypersensitivity
Rheumatoid arthritis	Serum sickness
Systemic lupus erythematosus	Drug allergy
Dermatomyositis	Amphetamine abuse
Rheumatic fever	
	Paraproteinaemias
Infections	Essential
	cryoglobulinaemia
Hepatitis B	Multiple myeloma
Acute respiratory infections	Macroglobulinaemia
Streptococcal infections	
Poststreptococcal glomerulonephritis	Others
Bacterial endocarditis	Dermal vasculitis
	Ulcerative colitis
Respiratory diseases	Cogan's syndrome
Loeffler's syndrome	Colon carcinoma
Asthma	
Serous otitis media	

1. Approach to Treatment

Excluding cases in which the cause of vasculitis is known (i.e. bacterial endocarditis or drug hypersensitivity) treatment is based on the ability to modify non-specifically the inflammatory response and in some cases to suppress the host immune system (Christian and Sergent, 1976). Many patients with vasculitis syndromes appear to have self-limited disease. The therapeutic goal is to suppress vascular inflammation during the period of active disease in the hope that irreversible damage to vital organs can be arrested or prevented.

2. Wegener's Granulomatosis

The most dramatic change in the natural history of vasculitis syndromes relates to Wegener's granulomatosis, where immunosuppressive therapy usually results in suppression of disease (Fauci and Wolff, 1973). In the majority of patients with Wegener's granulomatosis, the illness can be managed with immunosuppressive agents alone. Cyclophosphamide or azathioprine are employed in doses of 2 to 3mg/kg per day. Maintenance of therapy is influenced by signs of clinical activity and drug toxicity. Remission of Wegener's granulomatosis has been accomplished with several immunosuppressive drugs but some investigators have impressions that cyclophosphamide is the most effective.

In patients with very severe and acute manifestations of Wegener's granulomatosis, corticosteroid therapy is sometimes instituted along with immunosuppressive treatment. Prednisolone (or its equivalent) in doses of 1mg/kg/day (divided doses) are usually employed. When a remission ensues, prednisolone dosage should be gradually decreased and maintenance therapy attempted with the immunosuppressive agent.

3. Other Vasculitis Syndromes

With vasculitis syndromes other than Wegener's granulomatosis, management decisions are influenced by organ patterns of involvement. If there is evidence of significant renal disease, ischaemia of the gastrointestinal tract, cardiac involvement or major neurological disease, corticosteroid therapy in relatively large doses (i.e. prednisolone, 1mg/kg/day or more) is usually instituted. As in cases of systemic lupus erythematosus (chapter XIII), life compromising manifestations of vasculitis syndromes should be treated with corticosteroids in divided daily doses. A single daily dose or alternate day therapy, if they are to be employed at all, should be restricted to periods when disease activity is under control and where there are indications for lessened treatment. If the disease remits, the dose of prednisolone is reduced slowly over a period of weeks, while the patient is observed closely for evidence of recurrent activity of vasculitis. If corticosteroid therapy is not accompanied by a remission, cyclophosphamide or azathioprine therapy is sometimes initiated but, with the exception of Wegener's granulomatosis, the efficacy of immunosuppressive therapy has not been clearly established.

References and Recommended Reading

Christian, C.L. and Sergent, J.S.: Vasculitis syndromes: clinical and experimental models. American Journal of Medicine 61: 385 (1976).

Fauci, A.S. and Wolff, S.M.: Wegener's granulomatosis: studies in eighteen patients and a review of the literature. Medicine (Baltimore) 52: 535 (1973).

Sergent, J.S. and Christian, C.L.: Necrotising vasculitis after acute serous otitis media. Annals of Internal Medicine 81: 195 (1974).

Sergent, J.S.; Lockshin, M.D.; Christian, C.L. and Gocke, D.: Vasculitis with hepatitis B antigenemia: long-term observations in nine patients. Medicine (Baltimore) 55: 1 (1976).

Chapter XV

Dermatomyositis and Polymyositis

This chapter broadly describes therapeutic approaches which may be followed at present in the care of patients with dermatomyositis and polymyositis. As of now, these disorders have unknown aetiologies; there are no strictly agreed-upon criteria for their diagnosis, and their progression may be variable among groups of afflicted individuals. There is, consequently, room for disagreement about what constitutes the best in treatment. The discussion therefore, will try to accent the problems which need to be considered, as well as to summarise certain available modes of therapy (table I).

1. Diagnostic Considerations

Two features need highlighting: firstly, the diagnosis of disease, and secondly, the diagnosis of disease activity. It is not the purpose of this chapter to discuss the first, other than to stress the importance of obtaining as secure a diagnosis as possible before embarking on a treatment programme. In this connection, the presence of associated malignancy or other connective tissue disorder, such as progressive systemic sclerosis or Sjogren's syndrome, may alter the patient's prognosis.

Although certain special diagnostic methods, electromyography and muscle biopsy, are of great importance in initial evaluation, the diagnosis of disease activity and its response to therapy usually depends on elements of the patient's history, physical examination and laboratory tests. Exacerbations of disease may assume manifestations similar to the constellation of symptoms and signs which were present at the outset. Return of rash, telangectasia and arthralgia may be early indicators of exacerbation of illness. Return of weakness can be more difficult to evaluate, and other factors including complications of therapy, electrolyte imbalance or psychological reactions must be considered.

Table I. Outline of treatment of myositis

1. *Goals*
   a) Recovery of function
   b) Recovery of strength
   c) Return of laboratory abnormalities to normal

2. *Diagnostic Considerations*
   a) Disease type
   b) Disease activity

3. *Treatment*
   a) Physical measures
   b) Pharmacological agents
      i) Corticosteroids
      ii) Immunosuppressive agents (methotrexate, azathioprine, cyclophosphamide)

Laboratory findings, particularly increases in serum enzyme activities (creatinine phosphokinase, glutamic oxalacetic transaminase, and lactate dehydrogenase) and erythrocyte sedimentation rate may accompany exacerbations of inflammatory myopathy. In the chronically ill patient, however, these biochemical manifestations may be less marked than at the onset of disease. Active inflammation in muscle as well as vasculitis may be present, and continue in the absence of chemical evidence of active disease (Miller, 1973). In addition, changes in laboratory findings may not, in themselves, necessarily reflect changes in disease activity. Muscle trauma, injections, electromyographic studies, and exertion may lead to transient elevations of serum enzymes, unrelated to disease progression. Patients who assume full activities after a period of bed rest, or exercise programmes too taxing for their clinical states, may experience muscle aching along with enzyme elevations.

These brief remarks emphasise the need for analysis of changes in the patient's condition before deciding upon changes in the therapeutic programme.

2. Goals of Treatment

The goals of therapy must relate to the patient in a specific way and be clearly delineated and reconsidered as the course continues. Complete recovery of strength and the return of laboratory test results to normal are desirable goals in all patients. In some, they will not be attained. The clinician then must decide whether to consider these patients as treatment failures who require more, or different, medications, or to consider altering the goals he has set for them. In some patients, particularly those with life-threatening or rapidly progressing disease, it is usual to select the first option. In others, for example those with mild disease, it is possible to alter the goals to the limitation or halting of disease progression, and the maximisation of independent function.

The classification of treatment failures, then, is intrinsically related to the objectives of therapy. While it is recommended to attempt a complete reversal of abnormalities, this aim must be carefully weighed against the risks involved, and the chances of success.

3. Treatment

The major approach to treatment involves the use of drugs and physical measures and a spirit of understanding between clinician and patient which will allow a co-operative effort.

Rest during periods of active inflammation and physical therapy to rebuild muscle strength during periods of remission is indicated. Passive range of motion exercises to prevent contractures are important, particularly in children and in certain patients with overlap features of scleroderma, where contractures at the shoulder, elbow or around the ankle may rapidly develop. Despite daily therapy, however, contractures may progress in severely affected patients (Hill and Wood, 1970).

3.1 Corticosteroids

Corticosteroids are generally employed for the treatment of most patients. To the present, there have not been adequate controlled trials of their effectiveness, particularly since it has been pointed out that remissions occur spontaneously and several observers have found it difficult to demonstrate an influence on survival. Comparison of results among reported studies is difficult because of differences in their diagnostic criteria, time of onset of therapy in relation to disease onset, type of treatment and lack of matched comparison, or control groups. Nevertheless, corticosteroids have generally been considered beneficial, and are recommended for therapy in adults and children (Pearson, 1972; De Vere and Bradley, 1975).

In children, the aim of treatment is not to 'eradicate all manifestations of disease but to maintain patients in an ambulatory and independently functional state during the active stage of disease' (Rose, 1974). Similarly, Dubowitz (1976) suggested reduction in corticosteroid dosage in children as soon as clinical improvement was noted, without waiting for full clinical remission. He relied upon clinical findings rather than on serum enzyme determinations to indicate improvement.

In both adults and children, serious steroid complications have been encountered. Hypertension, cardiovascular decompensation, exacerbation of diabetes, active gastro-intestinal ulcer disease, sepsis, osteoporosis, as well as changes in appearance and psychological state have all been problems. The question of steroid myopathy has been more difficult to analyse, although several authorities have suggested that steroid-induced weakness may be a reason for the prolonged course of illness in some patients. It has also been suggested that some case reports advocating resort to immunosuppressive therapy in patients who failed to respond to corticosteroids may have related to this problem (Dubowitz, 1976).

The usual practice is to institute oral corticosteroid therapy in the range of 40 to 80mg of prednisolone per day for approximately 4 to 6 weeks until maximum benefit or remission of disease is achieved. The dose may then be very slowly and gradually reduced with careful monitoring of symptoms, physical findings and laboratory test results, to a lower or maintenance level in the range of 5 to 20mg. Other approaches are possible. Alternate day therapy has been used by some (DeVere and Bradley, 1975; Engle et al., 1971). Maintenance of corticosteroid therapy for the shortest possible period of time has also been advised (Dubowitz, 1976).

As pointed out above, there is no absolute yardstick other than the progress of one's own patient that can be best applied to monitoring of therapy. With this in mind, flexibility of approach, rather than rigid adherence to any one protocol of therapy may be best. There are occasional patients who demonstrate no clinical progression of disease after years of observation, with continued, intermittently elevated serum enzyme values not responsive to corticosteroid therapy. In these situations, one must ask whether the aim of therapy is to maintain independent and maximum function, or to strive for complete re-establishment of normal laboratory values.

Pearson (1972) has described several patterns of response to corticosteroid therapy in adults, which include:

1) A prompt decline in serum enzyme levels and return of strength in patients with disease of short duration, without malignancy, who have been treated early, usually within 2 months of disease onset.

2) A slower improvement in clinical and laboratory parameters among patients with more chronic illness, in whom strength is not fully regained.

3) Worsening and progression of illness after initial improvement in patients with malignancy and Sjogren's syndrome.

3.2 Immunosuppressive Agents

In certain circumstances, there may be a need to alter or add to corticosteroid treatment. This has usually occurred in 2 situations: (1) life-threatening, progressive illness without response to adequate corticosteroid therapy, or (2) partially responsive illness requiring large doses of steroids, where side-effects have become difficult to tolerate.

These circumstances have arisen with different frequencies in different series. To the present, it has been our experience that most patients with myositis, unassociated with malignancy or other disorders, can be treated with corticosteroids alone. However, there are a number of patients where this has not been so, and consideration may then be given to immunosuppressive therapy. Two general cautions should be introduced. The first deals with the lack of accurate, precise, and predictable information of the effect of these drugs in patients with myositis. Here, one confronts the same problems as mentioned with corticosteroid therapy (section 3.1), but in a less secure manner since experience with immunosuppressive agents is much more limited. The second deals with classifying these agents for the treatment of myositis as immunosuppressive. There is at present no compelling evidence that their immunosuppressive activity relates to their effectiveness, nor that any two of these agents operate in a similar manner or through similar mechanisms in inflammatory myopathy.

A number of agents have been used, including 6-mercaptopurine and chlorambucil, but most experience (still very small) has been with methotrexate, azathioprine and cyclophosphamide. Methotrexate was first employed in the treatment of dermatomyositis approximately 8 years ago (Malaviya et al., 1968) and since then there have been several reports indicating its usefulness, including a steroid-sparing effect, thus allowing reduction in corticosteroid dosage (Metzger et al., 1974). Methotrexate has been used intravenously, initially 10 to 15mg at intervals of 5 to 7 days with gradual increase to 30 to 50mg. After this, the frequency of administration is reduced to weekly, then biweekly and monthly. While few reports have described frequent severe side-effects in patients with myositis, toxicity was considered appreciable in a recent group of 5 patients (Arnett et al., 1973), 4 of whom had significant adverse effects. The most serious complication, methotrexate pneumonitis, occurred in 2 patients who had received oral therapy. Stomatitis was observed in 3 patients, hepatotoxicity in 1 and pruritus in another. At present, methotrexate is used intravenously in patients with myositis, since it undergoes more rapid excretion and may be less toxic when given in this manner (Malaviya et al., 1968). Other side-effects may include hepatotoxicity, suppression of bone marrow function, reduction in host defences against infection, gastrointestinal haemorrhage, dermatological toxicity, and nephropathy. Dysmorphogenicity is another area of concern.

Azathioprine (chapter III; sect. 3) has been added to corticosteroids with improvement noted in several small groups of patients. Doses used have varied but were in the range of 100 to 150mg/day orally during active disease, with a decrease to 50 to 75mg/day for maintenance therapy after disease remission had occurred. Major areas of toxicity of this agent are discussed in chapter III (sect. 3.3). One patient has been described with a hypersensitivity reaction to azathioprine which included muscle weakness and tenderness, which mimicked exacerbation of dermatomyositis (Goldenberg and Stor, 1975). Serum enzyme activities did not markedly change, however.

Cyclophosphamide has been used in few patients with myositis, thus far and results are inconclusive. The dose has not been completely evaluated, but a range of 100 to 200mg/day has been employed. Toxicity may involve depression of bone marrow function, increase in susceptibility to infection, alopecia, and haemorrhage from the urinary bladder.

4. Conclusion

Therapy in polymyositis and dermatomyositis still remains short of what is needed. Moreover, little data has thus far been accumulated about the proper use of immunosuppressive drugs. The question of their administration in children or in patients in their reproductive years also requires serious attention.

References and Recommended Reading

Arnett, F.C.; Whelton, J.C.; Zizic, T.M. and Stevens, M.B.: Methotrexate therapy in polymyositis. Annals of the Rheumatic Diseases 32: 536 (1973).

DeVere, R. and Bradley, W.G.: Polymyositis: Its presentation, morbidity and mortality. Brain 98: 637 (1975).

Dubowitz, V.: Treatment of dermatomyositis in childhood. Archives of Diseases in Childhood 51: 494 (1976).

Engle, W.K.; DeVivo, D.C.; Warmolts, J.R. and Schwartzman, R.J.: High-single-dose alternate-day prednisone (HSDAD-PRED) in neuromuscular disease. II International Congress on Muscle Diseases (Int. Cong. Series No. 273) Excerpta Medica, p.59 Amsterdam 1971.

Goldenberg, D.L. and Stor, R.A.: Azathioprine hypersensitivity mimicking an acute exacerbation of dermatomyositis. Journal of Rheumatology 2: 346 (1975).

Hill, R.H. and Wood, W.S.: Juvenile dermatomyositis. Canadian Medical Association Journal 103: 1152 (1970).

Malaviya, A.N.; Many, A. and Schwartz, R.S.: Treatment of dermatomyositis with methotrexate. Lancet 2: 485 (1968).

Metzger, A.L.; Bohan, A.; Goldberg, L.S.; Bluestone, R. and Pearson, C.M.: Polymyositis and dermatomyositis: combined methotrexate and corticosteroid therapy. Annals of Internal Medicine 81: 182 (1974).

Miller, J.J.: Late progression in dermatomyositis in childhood. Journal of Pediatrics 83: 543 (1973).

Pearson, C.M.: Polymyositis and dermatomyositis; in Hollander (Ed) Arthritis and Allied Conditions (Lea and Febiger, Philadelphia 1972).

Rose, A.L.: Childhood polymyositis. American Journal of Diseases of Children 127: 518 (1974).

Chapter XVI

Progressive Systemic Sclerosis

Progressive systemic sclerosis (PSS) is a generalised disorder of unknown aetiology involving the skin which also may affect the kidney, lungs, gastrointestinal tract, or other visceral organs. The early skin changes and joint stiffness may present a diagnostic problem, but the hide-bound skin and pinched facies characteristic of advanced PSS are easily recognised. Frequently, the disease is associated with a long, indolent course and nearly normal life span, but all too often it has a progressive course attended by renovascular, cardiopulmonary, or gastrointestinal decompensation.

Not only is the pathogenesis of progressive systemic sclerosis unknown, but also there is no consensus as to the genesis of the primary abnormality. Is the disease a vasculitic syndrome, the result of abnormal collagen synthesis, or is it of immunological origin? There are few other diseases about which such fundamental questions remain unanswered. Raynaud's phenomenon, telangiectasias, renal vascular hypertension, pulmonary hypertension, and probably most of the visceral manifestations of progressive systemic sclerosis attest to vascular abnormalities. Altered collagen is readily apparent as sclerotic and atrophied skin. Positive antinuclear antibodies (particularly with a speckled pattern), occasional positive tests for rheumatoid factor, and alterations in immunoglobulin levels are manifestations of immunological abnormalities.

1. Goals of Treatment

There is currently no cure for progressive systemic sclerosis. No medication has been proven to be of unequivocal efficacy. Drugs are used for the treatment and relief of symptoms, but treatment also involves physical therapy, occupational counselling and psychological support in order that the patient may continue to function as well as possible.

Treatment is directed at two aspects of the condition: (1) the associated medical problems, and (2) the disease process itself. The first category of treatment involves standard modes of therapy directed toward medical problems which patients with progressive systemic sclerosis share in common with many other patients: hypertension, congestive heart failure, pulmonary insufficiency, oesophagitis and pain, to name a few. These standard treatments will not be commented on except for emphasis in certain instances.

The second category of treatment is that which is given with some theoretical rationale in an attempt to modify the disease process itself. In contrast to the first aspect of treatment, there is very little that is standard. Many drugs have been employed, but reported results vary widely. The long and variable course of the disease, the absence of a laboratory test which accurately parallels disease activity, and the frequent lack of adequate control groups, makes the assessment of these reports of treatment difficult. Response to treatment, or lack of it, probably depends as much on the stage of the disease being treated as the drug employed. Drugs used in the management of progressive systemic sclerosis may be classified as vasoactive, anti-inflammatory and experimental. The following sections deal with these drugs and the cautions which should be observed in their use.

2. Vasoactive Drugs

The drugs listed in table I may increase the threshold to vasospasm (Varadi and Lawrence, 1969), but there is no evidence that they alter the course of the disease. Their clinical efficacy has not been well documented in controlled trials. These agents are sometimes employed empirically, with the reasoning that in usual doses they can do little harm. However, the doses needed to produce symptomatic relief may be high and side-effects frequent. Failure to respond to one agent does not preclude the use of another; the dosages may have to be increased in the winter and decreased in the summer. In rare instances, vasoactive drugs may result in an exacerbation of symptoms; this is presumably due to a 'steal syndrome' in which unaffected vessels dilate normally and drain blood from areas supplied by sclerotic vessels which are no longer able to dilate physiologically.

Because the digital ulcerations associated with Raynaud's phenomenon present such a difficult management problem, vasoactive drugs have been employed in an attempt to ameliorate vascular spasm and increase digital blood flow, but effects are not long-lasting. Thus, intra-arterial reserpine currently has no generally accepted indication: it may be used once or twice in the management of Raynaud's phenomenon with severe digital ulceration with the expectation that its efficacy will probably last between several days and several months. Surgical sympathectomy may be viewed in a similar light; it increases peripheral blood flow initially but has a limited long-term effect (Winkelmann et al., 1971).

Table I. Vasoactive drugs used in the management of scleroderma

Reserpine	0.25mg to 1.0mg orally 4 times daily 0.5mg to 1.0mg intra-arterially
Methyldopa	500 to 2000mg orally 4 times daily
Guanethidine	10 to 50mg orally 4 times daily

3. Antihypertensive Drug Therapy

Hypertension is generally due to either generalised atherosclerosis or to intimal hyperplasia characteristic of scleroderma. As it is frequently associated with high renin levels, antihypertensive drugs which inhibit renin release such as propranolol, clonidine, methyldopa, reserpine, and ganglion blockers may be useful. Diuretic treatment increases plasma renin levels and may aggravate renal disease.

The appearance of malignant hypertension with its associated end organ damage, presages rapid deterioration of clinical condition and irreversible renal failure. Intravenous sodium nitroprusside, diazoxide, or other equally potent hypotensive agents can be employed to bring the blood pressure under control as quickly as possible. Failing this, dialysis or renal transplantation should be considered, if such services can be arranged and if visceral manifestations other than renovascular disease are not in themselves life-compromising. There is a general impression that the toxic state, sometimes associated with accelerated hypertension, is an indication for bilateral nephrectomy, but this has not been evaluated systematically.

4. Anti-inflammatory Drugs

The scleroedematous phase of progressive systemic sclerosis, joint pain and stiffness, and myositis are manifestations of widespread inflammation. Treatment is tailored to symptoms. There is no evidence that prolonged or high-dose anti-inflammatory treatment will alter the course of the disease. However, when used judiciously, anti-inflammatory drugs such as aspirin or corticosteroids can unquestionably improve the quality of a patient's life.

Aspirin may provide symptomatic relief when used in moderate dosage (600 to 2400mg daily). There is no controlled trial on the use of antimalarial agents, but their anti-inflammatory properties are useful in the treatment of chronic cutaneous manifestations of systemic lupus erythematosus (chapter XIII; sect. 1.1) and treatment of patients with progressive systemic sclerosis having positive tests for antinuclear antibodies has been reported (Winkelmann et al., 1971).

The only generally accepted role for corticosteroid or ACTH treatment in progressive systemic sclerosis is in the management of severe myositis. Doses of 40 to 60mg daily of prednisolone may be used early and then gradually reduced over several weeks or months. This has not been demonstrated to alter the long-term course of the disease, but may occasionally provide short-term benefit as discussed in chapter XV on myositis (sect. 3.1). Corticosteroid treatment has not been demonstrated to affect progressive cardiac, gastrointestinal, or pulmonary manifestations and it may exacerbate hypertension. Low dose corticosteroid therapy (i.e. 5mg prednisolone per day) may improve such constitutional symptoms as weight loss, decreased appetite and fatigue, but leave the clinician with the unhappy alternative of long-term treatment or reducing steroid dosage in the face of progressive disease.

5. Experimental Agents

The list of experimental drugs tried for the treatment of scleroderma is long. Many were first reported with good results but none has withstood long-term scrutiny. Currently, D-penicillamine and colchicine on the basis of their effect on experimental models, have the best theoretical rationale for use but their efficacy has not been proved.

Penicillamine chelates copper and other heavy metals and interferes with intermolecular cross-linking of collagen. It results in increased amounts of young, soluble collagen and may accelerate the turnover of pre-existing insoluble collagen, presumably by cleaving intermolecular bands. If given to patients with Wilson's disease or growing animals, it produces fragile skin; but visceral collagen may have different cross-links than cutaneous collagen (Davis and Bleehen, 1976). The side-effects of penicillamine are potentially serious (chapter III; sect. 2.3) and its efficacy has not been demonstrated in controlled trials.

Colchicine *in vitro* decreases the collagen output of fibroblasts and increases collagen degradation; rats made cirrhotic with carbon tetrachloride showed an improvement in liver function tests and a decrease in liver fibrosis when treated with colchicine. Initial favourable results, including decreased dermal collagen in some patients (Alarcon-Segovia et al., 1974) have not been reproduced (Guttadauria et al., 1976).

The use of para-aminobenzoic acid (Potaba) was first reported in 1953 and was felt to soften skin and promote the healing of digital ulcers. This has not been substantiated. Doses of more than 6 to 8g daily are associated with nausea, vomiting, pruritus, drug rash, drug fever, gastrointestinal toxicity, and toxic hepatitis. Two cases of agranulocytosis have been reported.

Dimethylsulphoxide (DMSO), a chemical with multiple industrial uses, is absorbed readily through the skin. When applied locally in scleroderma it may lead to softening and healing of digital ulcers. Toxicity appears minimal, but studies are uncontrolled. A recent symposium covers many aspects of this treatment (Fleischmajer, 1975).

The striking predominance of scleroderma in females prompted a trial of testosterone in the early 1950s, but results were limited. D-Thyroxine treatment was evaluated in the few doubleblind controlled studies in scleroderma research but was not effective. Relaxin, an extract of the ovaries of pregnant sows which relaxes the pubic symphysis prior to parturition, in an uncontrolled trial was thought to promote loosening of the skin and healing of scleroderma ulcers. Low molecular weight dextran, a 'desludging' agent which decreases blood viscosity and increases capillary flow, has been advocated but its efficacy in affecting skin temperature was not confirmed. Benefit is claimed for griseofulvin but the study was uncontrolled. Both thioguanine and azathioprine have been used without success.

6. Symptomatic Measures

Even though no single drug has proven efficacy in treatment of progressive systemic sclerosis, rational management is of great importance because of the potentially long survival of these patients. Environmental, personal, and occupational guidance may make the difference between a tolerable and a miserable existence. An ambient temperature of 25°C (78°F) is recommended, although this may not be achieved by a move to the tropics because of ubiquitous air conditioning. Patients should dress warmly, since Raynaud's phenomenon may be precipitated by either central or peripheral cooling. Activities involving manual dexterity or finger tip friction are best avoided; gloves both protect and warm the hands. Lubricating oils and creams are often used empirically. If digital ulcerations develop, antibiotic creams, acid fuchsin, gentian violet, and continuous wet dermatological dressings have been employed with varying success. Vasoconstrictor drugs such as amphetamines, nicotine, and ergotamine are contraindicated.

Malabsorption which may be due in part to bacterial overgrowth should be recorded by the clinician. It is sometimes helped by courses of tetracycline (250g qid) or ampicillin (500g qid). Reflux oesophagitis is so common that measures are best taken early to prevent its occurrence. Coffee, tea, tobacco and other stimulants of gastrin production are best avoided. If symptoms of oesophagitis are present, patients should have no food within 2 to 4 hours of bedtime and begin an intensive regimen of antacid therapy. Elevation of the head of the bed on 6-inch blocks may prevent some reflux at night-time.

References and Recommended Reading

Alarcon-Segovia, D.; Ibanez, G.; Kershenobich, D. and Rojkind, M.: Treatment of scleroderma (letter). Lancet 1: 1054 (1974).

Davis, P. and Bleehen, S.S.: D-penicillamine in the treatment of rheumatoid arthritis and progressive systemic sclerosis. British Journal of Dermatology 94 (6): 705 (1976).

Fleischmajer, R.: Discussion of paper: Methodology and techniques in the evaluation of dimethyl sulfoxide for connective tissue disorders. Annals of the New York Academy of Science 243: 393 (1975).

Guttadauria, M.; Diamond, H.; Kaplan, D.: Colchicine in the treatment of scleroderma. (Abstract). ARA National Meeting, December 9, 1976.

LeRoy, E.C.; Downey, J.A. and Cannon, P.J.: Skin capillary blood flow in scleroderma. Journal of Clinical Investigation 50: 930 (1971).

Pettinger, W.A. and Mitchell, H.C.: Minoxidil — an alternative to nephrectomy for refractory hypertension. New England Journal of Medicine 289: 167 (1973).

Tuffanelli, D.L.: A clinical trial with dimethylsulfoxide in scleroderma. Archives of Dermatology (Chicago) 93: 724 (1966).

Varadi, D.P. and Lawrence, A.M.: Suppression of Raynaud's phenomenon by methyldopa. Archives of Internal Medicine 124: 13 (1969).

Winkelmann, R.K.; Kierland, R.R.; Perry, H.D.; Muller, S.A. and Sams, W.M.: Management of scleroderma. Mayo Clinic Proceedings 46: 128 (1971).

Chapter XVII

Infective Arthropathies

In the infective arthropathies one, or sometimes more than one, of a number of infective organisms has reached the joint tissues; usually from the blood stream, but sometimes from adjacent bone or skin, from broken down infected rheumatoid nodules over pressure points, or from foreign bodies introduced into the joint from outside (e.g. thorns, metal fragments, needles and various therapeutic agents). Devitalised inflamed tissues in devitalised patients, such as rheumatoid joints in rheumatoid subjects, are more likely to become infected than normal joints in normal people, whatever the source of infection. Although many different types of infective agents may cause arthritis, only the septic pyarthroses are considered here.

1. Septic Arthritis (pyarthrosis)

To confirm the diagnosis, the joint is aspirated and the fluid examined for bacteria and cultured. Blood cultures may also be set up and should always be done if there is fever, systemic upset, rigor or other evidence of disseminated infection. Although infecting organisms should always be tested for drug sensitivity, treatment should not be delayed to await bacteriological results. Empirical treatment (see below) is started promptly on the basis of the most likely organism(s) and then changed to the most appropriate antimicrobial agent(s), once the results of sensitivity tests are known.

The joint fluid usually demonstrates a high leucocytosis but white blood cell counts do not always show a leucocytosis. The most common organism infecting joint tissues is *Staphylococcus aureus* (particularly when superimposed on rheumatoid arthritis), but *Streptococcus pyogenes, faecalis* or *viridans* are occasionally found and sometimes the gonococcus, pneumococcus, meningococcus, *Haemophilus influenzae, Escherichia coli, Brucella abortus* or *melitensis* and a number of other organisms. Tuberculous infection of bone or joint should never be forgotten (see section 2), and anaerobic infections may easily be missed, unless special cultures are set up to grow these organisms.

1.1 General Approach to Treatment

Treatment depends on the invading organism and the response to therapy, but in general the patient with a pyarthrosis is rested in bed, the joint immobilsed, sometimes in plaster of Paris, and sometimes put onto traction. Therapy should not be delayed to await the results of joint or blood cultures but should be initiated early on the basis of a hopefully inspired hunch, which depends essentially on the case history, evidence of infection elsewhere and the probabilities of a particular infection being present.

The smear from the joint fluid may demonstrate Gram positive or negative cocci, which may give a lead to therapy, but if no organism is seen on smears in an adult patient, or a Gram negative coccus is seen, benzylpenicillin may be given 50,000 to 75,000 units per kg 6-hourly intravenously or by continuous intravenous drip. Penicillin rapidly penetrates the joints. An alternative is ampicillin, 50mg/kg intravenously or intramuscularly 6-hourly. Infections due to gonococci, pneumococci or sensitive staphylococci will probably respond satisfactorily, but unfortunately many strains of *Staphylococcus aureus*, the most common invader, are insensitive to these agents.

Newman (1976) in a recent review of the treatment of different types of septic arthritis over the last 30 years at the Nuffield Orthopaedic Centre in Oxford, noted that in the first decade that 29% of organisms were penicillin resistant, compared with 59% in the last decade. Nevertheless, Kellgren and his colleagues in 1958 in Manchester, in their original description of septic arthritis occurring as a complication in rheumatoid arthritis, found that only 3 of 10 strains of *Staphylococcus aureus* isolated were penicillin sensitive. In a study of 77 cases of pyarthrosis occurring in the native population of Nigeria between 1973 and 1976, knees and hips were most commonly involved; in 59% of cases by *Staph. aureus*, 22% by mixed organisms, 11% by *Klebsiella* spp, and 7% by streptococci. In 65.5% of cases, staphylococci were resistant to penicillin (Sturrock, pers. comm. 1977).

For the above reasons, flucloxacillin 250mg 6-hourly intramuscularly (or alternative penicillinase-resistant penicillin) may therefore be preferred initially, later continued at the same dosage by mouth when the infection has been brought under control. Alternatives are combinations of flucloxacillin and ampicillin (250mg of each by intramuscular injection 6-hourly), or ampicillin and cloxacillin (250 to 500mg of each 4 to 6-hourly intramuscularly or intravenously), diethanolamine fusidate (by intravenous infusion) or sodium fusidate (500mg 8-hourly with meals by mouth). Mitchell and his colleagues (1976) believe that neither benzylpenicillin nor ampicillin should ever be used to treat staphylococcal infections, and although they favour gentamicin they prefer to keep this drug in reserve because of its tendency to cause ototoxicity, preferring cloxacillin and fusidic acid initially.

Because of the high mortality in septic arthritis intravenous or intramuscular administration is preferred initially. Although single intra-articular injections of one or several antibiotics may prove helpful initially, since these agents reach the joint effectively given systemically and as intra-articular injections of antibiotics may cause an annoying painful and persistent synovitis, most clinicians prefer to avoid intra-articular medication (e.g. Newman, 1976; Russel and Ansell, 1972). Most orthopaedic surgeons favour surgical drainage. Gristina et al. (1974) in staphylococcal septic arthritis, which is most common in knees in rheumatoid arthritics, favour arthrotomy with drainage or through and through irrigation with fluid containing the appropriate antibiotic rather than repeated needle aspirations. Goldenberg and his colleagues (1975), however, found no superiority of surgical drainage over needle aspiration in the treatment of a mixed group of septic arthropathies.

When cultures are available and drug sensitivities are known, if progress is unsatisfactory therapy should be changed to the most appropriate agent. It must be emphasised that *early diagnosis and treatment is essential,* for later therapy means a higher mortality and cases of septic arthritis are easily missed, particularly in rheumatoid arthritis.

Any local exacerbation in 1 or 2 joints, particularly if the joints are hot and the patient febrile should be investigated as a possible case of septic arthritis, rather than treated as a local exacerbation of rheumatoid disease. Delay may be dangerous, mortality averaging around 30% in such cases.

1.2 Specific Plan of Antibacterial Therapy

A plan of bacteriological warfare suggested by Brian Lacey, Professor of Bacteriology at Westminster Hospital, London, is as follows:

1) Aspirate the joint (e.g. the knee). If it is cloudy, but not viscous, send the fluid to the laboratory for immediate examination and culture and give benzylpenicillin 2 mega units, cloxacillin 0.5g and, separately, gentamicin 80mg intramuscularly 6-hourly; providing there are no contraindications such as known hypersensitivity, impaired renal function or disease of the 8th cranial nerve. Gentamicin is particularly liable to cause ototoxicity in the elderly, in those with impaired renal function and in patients in whom other potentially ototoxic agents have been used previously (neomycin, streptomycin, kanamycin, tobramycin). Many would, however, prefer to omit gentamicin from this initial therapy because of this risk, but even with poor renal function gentamicin may still be given if care is taken to adjust the dose suitably (with or without the help of a nomogram) and to monitor serum concentrations at 24 to 48 hour intervals.

If the aspirated fluid is cloudy and viscous or clots, give the 3 antibiotics as above and possibly 1 injection only into the joint of 0.25 mega units of benzylpenicillin,

20mg cloxacillin and 10mg gentamicin. Repeated intra-articular injections are likely to provoke a persistent synovitis and many clinicians prefer to avoid intra-articular injections of antibiotic altogether.

2) Review at 3 to 6 hours in the light of the immediate laboratory results, especially microscopy for bacteria or pus cells, immunology (antibody) tests for bacterial antigens and possibly glucose content, which is reduced with bacterial infection.

3) Review in 48 hours in the light of the clinical state, bacteriological, culture and sensitivity results and possibly, radiological changes. Gentamicin dosage would now usually be reduced to 80mg 8-hourly. Serum levels of gentamicin and other agents should be requested if needed. Re-aspiration is then usually performed or surgical drainage considered.

4) Continue on chosen antibiotic for a further 10 to 14 days, and

5) Continue on oral antibiotics for a further 6 to 12 weeks.

These are suggestions only. One cannot generalise, for 1 patient may have a mild local gonococcal pyarthrosis, in another the infected joint is merely one manifestation of diffuse pyaemia in an ill debilitated rheumatoid arthritic who proves at autopsy to have abscesses in many parts of the body. The rheumatoid arthritic with the worst prognoses are:

a) The debilitated, ill, seropositive, nodular cases, particularly the very crippled bed-fast sufferers.
b) Those on high dosage long-standing corticosteroid therapy.
c) Patients with Felty's syndrome.
d) Those with other infected foci elsewhere imperfectly controlled.

When the infection is controlled, it is clearly wise to continue treatment for several weeks on the appropriate antibiotic by mouth, or relapses may occur. Russell and Ansell (1972) maintained such therapy in their series of cases for 6 to 12 weeks subsequently. Surgical drainage was only performed in 2 complicated cases, the average number of joint aspirations being 3, done at 24 to 48 hour intervals and the initial high dosage antibiotic intravenous therapy was maintained for 2 full weeks.

2. Tuberculous Arthritis

Infection of a joint or spine with *Mycobacterium tuberculosis* was once common in Great Britain, then it became rare and now, although still uncommon, it has to be thought of when any odd, unusual arthropathy is seen. Biopsies of joint tissue may resemble rheumatoid and other arthropathies. Histologically, cultures for *M. tuberculosis* should always be done in doubtful cases. Spine and hips are the most commonly involved, knee, ankle, foot and sacroiliac less commonly. Joints are initially rested, possibly with daily passive movement to maintain mobility and traction or splintage to correct or prevent deformity. The spine is initially immobilised in a plaster bed for at least 3 weeks. Surgery may involve debridement and fusion of the spine or debridement of other joints.

The main danger in the treatment of tuberculous involvement of bone and joint is, as with the treatment of any other tuberculous condition, the emergence of resistant strains of bacilli. It is for this reason that the drugs used are given in combination, the most effective initial combinations being: (1) streptomycin + isoniazid + rifampicin, and (2) ethambutol + isoniazid + rifampicin.

Until sensitivities are known, streptomycin, rifampicin and isoniazid should be started. It is rare to use today the high dose of isoniazid of some years ago, when, with doses exceeding 300mg daily of isoniazid, 50 to 100mg of pyridoxine had to be given to prevent peripheral neuritis. Dosage is now 3mg/kg daily, i.e. an average of 200mg daily in divided dosage. Patients who metabolise the drug rapidly (fast acetylators) may need larger doses (5mg/kg daily).

Streptomycin is given intramuscularly. It diffuses into most body tissues including synovial fluid. The usual dose is 0.5 to 1g intramuscularly daily, depending on age and weight. When the patient is over age 40 or there is evidence of renal insufficiency, streptomycin must be given on alternate days and the dosage should be monitored by serum streptomycin levels. High blood levels and early ototoxic reactions occur in the presence of impaired renal function, as streptomycin is excreted unchanged by the kidneys. The vestibular branch of the 8th nerve may be affected, with vertigo, nausea, vomiting and ataxia, which can be permanent. Rifampicin is usually well tolerated and is given in a dosage of 10mg/kg (around 600mg daily). Because of risk of hepatotoxicity, its use in alcoholics and patients with liver disease is best avoided.

Treatment should continue for 12 months. In severe disseminated disease, it is wise to use streptomycin in full dosage initially daily, reducing dosage after 2 to 3 months to twice a week for a further 2 to 4 months. Surgical measures should be deferred until the infection is controlled, usually after 3 to 4 weeks.

References and Recommended Reading

Goldenberg, D.L.; Brandt, K.D.; Cohen, A.S. and Cathcart, E.S.: Treatment of septic arthritis. Comparison of needle aspiration and surgery as initial modes of joint drainage. Arthritis and Rheumatism 18: 83 (1975).

Gristina, A.G.; Rovere, G.D. and Shoji, H.: Spontaneous septic arthritis complicating rheumatoid arthritis. Journal of Bone and Joint Surgery 56A: 1180 (1974).

Kellgren, J.H.; Ball, J.; Fairbrother, R.W. and Barnes, K.L.: Suppurative arthritis complicating rheumatoid arthritis. British Medical Journal 1: 1193 (1958).

Mitchell, W.S.; Brooks, P.M.; Stevenson, R.D. and Buchanan, W.W.: Septic arthritis in patients with rheumatoid disease: a still underdiagnosed complication. Journal of Rheumatology 3: 124 (1976).

Newman, J.H.: Review of septic arthritis throughout the antibiotic era. Annals of the Rheumatic Diseases 35: 198 (1976).

Russell, A.S. and Ansell, B.M.: Septic arthritis. Annals of the Rheumatic Diseases 31: 40 (1972).

Chapter XVIII

Rheumatic Fever

Rheumatic fever classically develops some 10 to 18 days after a throat infection with streptococci of group A haemolytic type. Although heralding the disease, fever and arthritis are not of serious import; it is the carditis which is the problem. As yet, no therapy has been shown to influence the course of the disease so that both aspirin and corticosteroids must be considered as merely palliative therapy (Markovitz and Kuttner, 1965).

1. Initial Treatment

Once a diagnosis of rheumatic fever has been made, the elimination of streptococci is essential. The drug of choice is benzylpenicillin and this should be given as 1 mega unit a day for a minimum of 10 days. In patients sensitive to penicillin, erythromycin 250mg 4 times daily for a total of 10 days can be given. Following this, prophylactic therapy (section 2) should be instituted.

Aspirin in adequate dosage of 100mg/kg a day has a dramatic effect on both fever and joint symptoms. However, if there is pre-existing carditis or severe carditis has already developed in this attack, high dosage salicylate therapy can cause further cardiac embarrassment (Bywaters and Thomas, 1961). There is little doubt that corticosteroids do control the acute exudative phase of rheumatic carditis, but neither the 1 or 5 year result in the USA/UK study (1960) showed any significant difference between these three treatment groups; namely aspirin, ACTH or cortisone. It has been suggested that in this study, therapy was too short, but the results of the combined rheumatic fever study (1960) using 12 weeks of prednisone showed no difference between the corticosteroid and aspirin groups. Dorfmann and his colleagues' results in 1961 may well have been due to the inclusion of cases with mild carditis, as the prognosis for these is excellent.

Thus, in general, in patients with no or minimal carditis (i.e. prolongation of the PR interval or a soft apical systolic murmur), aspirin should be used, but if the patient already has serious carditis, particularly with established mitral valve disease and enlargement of the left ventricle, a corticosteroid such as prednisolone is better therapy. It should be given in a dosage of 2mg/kg body weight a day. If the patient is in congestive cardiac failure, supportive therapy with diuretics should be given early. Digitalis can be added, if required, once the inflammatory element has been brought under control with corticosteroids. In general, both prednisolone and aspirin will probably need to be continued in full dosage for 4 to 6 weeks and then gradually tailed off. The rebound phenomenon has occurred more frequently with corticosteroids than with aspirin, but the exact significance of this is uncertain and it may merely represent persistent disease activity.

2. Prophylactic Therapy

While there is good evidence that prompt administration of antibiotics for streptococcal infection reduces the incidence of rheumatic fever, there is no such good evidence that once the patient has had an attack of rheumatic fever, treatment of streptococcal attacks reduces the incidence of second attacks. However, prophylactic therapy does prevent further attacks (Evans, 1950; Feinstein, 1964). This may be carried out in several ways. The first studies were done with sulphonamides, and sulphadiazine 1g daily is certainly an effective means of preventing further group A haemolytic streptococcal infections. In patients with established heart disease there is a slight preference for sulphonamide rather than penicillin so as to minimise the risk of the development of subacute bacterial endocarditis with penicillin-resistant organisms. However, most patients are currently maintained on penicillin prophylaxis which can either be by oral penicillin 250mg twice daily or benzathine penicillin intramuscularly given as 1.2 mega units once a month. Both are equally satisfactory.

Only very rarely does penicillin cause hypersensitivity, the most usual sign being urticaria or some other type of rash. Very occasionally, more serious reactions have been noted, particularly after intramuscular injection, which can also cause some pain at the site of injection. If penicillin sensitivity occurs, prophylaxis with erythromycin 125mg twice daily may be considered.

Recurrences are most likely in the first year after an attack, so prophylaxis is mandatory for the first few years. It is important, however, to realise that recurrences of rheumatic fever can occur at any age, even in adult life, and that they tend to mimic each other, so that if carditis has occurred in the first attack it will also recur in subsequent ones. It has therefore become customary to suggest that in patients with residual carditis, prophylaxis should be given indefinitely. The danger period appears to be the teenage years when prophylactic medication is often forgotten, so reinforcement instruction on importance of medication compliance is constantly required.

Should streptococcal infection occur despite the patient being on a prophylactic regimen, this should be promptly and vigorously treated with full therapeutic dosage of penicillin given for a minimum of 10 days or, if the patient is sensitive to penicillin, erythromycin 250mg 4 times daily for 10 days.

3. Prevention of Bacterial Endocarditis

Bacteremia from tooth extraction and other oral surgical procedures such as manipulation of periodontal tissues, as well as removal of tonsils and adenoids and the instrumentation of the genitourinary tract, can cause bacterial endocarditis in patients who already have residual damage to heart valves. The purpose therefore of prophylactic antibiotics before such procedures is that they will prevent the bacteremia, or, should it occur, reduce its magnitude and duration.

Penicillin remains the drug of choice for dental treatment or operations on the tonsils and adenoids. Intramuscular penicillin should be given for 1 to 2 hours before the procedure is carried out and continued in full dosage for a minimum of 48 hours. The dosage before operations should be intramuscular, but provided the patient is cooperative the postoperative doses can be by mouth. Erythromycin can be given in cases of penicillin sensitivity. For instrumentation of the genitourinary tract, it is usual to add streptomycin 50mg/kg, not to exceed 1g daily, for 48 hours; again beginning approximately 1 hour before the procedure.

References and Recommended Reading

Bywaters, E.G.L. and Thomas, G.T.: Bed rest, salicylate and steroid in rheumatic fever. British Medical Journal 1: 1628 (1961).

Combined Rheumatic Fever Study Group: A comparison of the effect of prednisone and acetyl salicylic acid on the incidence of residual rheumatic heart disease. New England Journal of Medicine 262: 895 (1960).

Dorfman, A.; Gross, J.L. and Lorniez, A.E.: The treatment of acute rheumatic fever. Paediatrics 27: 692 (1961).

Evans, J.A.P.: Discussion on the management of rheumatic fever and its oral complications; oral penicillin in prophylaxis of streptococcal and rheumatic fever relapse. Proceedings of the Royal Society of Medicine 43: 206 (1950).

Feinstein, A.R.; Wood, H.H.; Spagnuolo, M.; Taranta, A.; Tursky, E. and Kleinberg, E.: Oral prophylaxis of recurrent rheumatic fever. Sulphadiazine versus a double daily dose of penicillamine. Journal of the American Medical Association 188: 489 (1964).

Markowitz, M. and Kuttner, A.G.: Rheumatic Fever. Diagnosis, Management and Prevention, Vol. 2 Major Problems in Clinical Paediatrics (Saunders, Philadelphia 1965).

UK and US Joint Report: The evolution of rheumatic heart disease in children. Five year report on the co-operative clinical trial of ACTH, cortisone and aspirin. Circulation 22: 503 (1960).

Chapter XIX

Juvenile Chronic Polyarthritis

The basic rule in treatment is to administer those agents for which the demonstrated value is greater than the threat of serious toxicity, unless serious complications are present. Many children with chronic polyarthritis do not complain of pain, but protective muscle spasm is usually present around involved joints. In such circumstances a non-steroidal anti-inflammatory analgesic should be employed. In general, therapy should be continued for several months after the active disease process has subsided, and even then withdrawal should be extremely cautious.

1. General Approach to Treatment

In selecting the type of drug, one is influenced by the pattern of disease process present. Thus, in serious systemic illness high dose aspirin is used immediately, followed, if necessary, by another potent non-steroidal anti-inflammatory analgesic, such as indomethacin. If these fail, the early use of corticosteroids or corticotrophin will have to be considered. Conversely, with a single joint, particularly if there is little pain or spasm, simple analgesics on a self-demand regimen can be given.

As the prognosis of seropositive juvenile rheumatoid arthritis, both in respect of continuing activity and joint destruction, is so much more serious than in seronegative disease, the advisability of introducing 'specific' antirheumatic drugs such as gold or penicillamine needs to be considered much earlier. Whether disease patterns respond differently is not known, and it may well be that those young patients, usually male, who have a pauci-articular arthritis, and ultimately develop sacroiliitis, will do better on indomethacin, phenylbutazone or naproxen than on aspirin. Thus, in selecting appropriate drug therapy for an individual case it is extremely important to assess the type of disease present. It should also be appreciated that the drug therapy is but one part of the management of children suffering from chronic polyarthritis (Bywaters, 1976; Ansell, 1975).

2. Non-Steroidal Anti-inflammatory Analgesics

2.1 Aspirin

Aspirin is still the most valuable drug in the management of this disorder, as it can relieve fever and joint pain, and children tolerate it well. There are many preparations available. While older children can swallow tablets, soluble preparations are better for young patients, and, provided the timing and dosage is appropriate to the medication employed, round-the-clock suppression of disease activity can usually be achieved. In general, it is desirable to try and maintain the serum salicylate level, midway between doses near 2.2mmol/L (30mg/100ml). When this is done, it is unlikely that serious hepatotoxicity will occur. In our own experience (Russell et al., 1971), abnormal levels of transaminases were not recorded unless blood levels were particularly high. Despite these abnormal transaminases, serious liver impairment has not been recorded in children (Rich and Johnson, 1973; Athreya, 1975).

The dosage of salicylate should be of the order of 80mg/kg body weight per day, although Makela (1975) suggests $2g/m^2$. In children with serious systemic illness it may be necessary to increase the dosage to 100 or 200mg/kg per day for short periods to bring the disease under control. In such circumstances, the child should be observed closely for the first evidence of salicylism — over-breathing, vomiting or drowsiness. If one of these occurs, or if this dosage is continued for more than a week, a blood salicylate level should be performed. It is important to remember that children rarely complain of tinnitus or deafness.

Once the acute systemic phase has passed the dosage of salicylate should be reduced to maintain control. When the child is well enough to return to school the question of divided daily dosage may prove a problem. It is therefore with this in mind that we undertook studies on benorylate, a chemical combination of aspirin and paracetamol (acetaminophen) in order to control the disease process and maintain function (and get satisfactory salicylate levels) it was found necessary to give approximately 200mg/kg body weight of benorylate per day. This can still be given as a twice daily dosage, which is of great advantage to the parents of the school-child, who then do not have to send a mid-day dose to school. As the paracetamol (acetaminophen) level appears to parallel the salicylate level, monitoring salicylate levels is all that is necessary (Powell et al., 1974).

2.2 Indomethacin

The initial report of sudden death occurring in 2 children receiving indomethacin (Jacobs, 1967) was extremely disturbing. However, these children had received multiple drugs and it was difficult to be certain that indomethacin was the actual cause of their demise. Initial studies at the MRC Rheumatism Unit at Taplow, where we had undertaken a comparative study of indomethacin (2.5mg/kg daily in divided doses) and aspirin (80mg daily) continued. During these studies, indomethacin was shown to be as effective as aspirin in controlling joint symptoms, and of value in suppressing fever. Further studies on tolerance have shown it to be a valuable drug, both in cases which have failed to respond to aspirin and in those where reduction of corticosteroid dosage is desirable.

Although we have used up to 2.5mg/kg daily, in general our dosage has tended to be somewhat lower and in the main it has been given in divided doses. For children who are particularly slow, or appear to their parents to be stiff in the mornings, the use of a moderate sized night dose has been extremely valuable in relieving morning stiffness. Indeed, indomethacin at night, often in the form of a suspension, which is particularly valuable in paediatric practice, and full salicylate dosage by day has proved a satisfactory combination. Side-effects are similar to those seen in adults (chapter II; sect. 4.4), although the complaints of dizziness and headaches are relatively rare. Recurrent vomiting and loss of appetite, particularly in young children, have proved to be the main problem with indomethacin therapy. The more usual gastrointestinal complaints, including haematemesis, have been seen, usually in referred cases on a much higher dose than that suggested here.

2.3 Ibuprofen

A comparative study of ibuprofen (20mg/kg daily) with aspirin (80mg/kg daily) has shown it to be of similar potency with respect to control of joint symptoms and maintenance of function, with minimal side-effects. Subsequently, particularly in 'difficult to treat' cases and during tolerance studies, it has proved to be a useful drug (Ansell, 1973). Fever was not controlled at doses of 20mg/kg daily but studies are in progress in the USA at doses of 40mg/kg daily, at which level it may well be more valuable for fever. It is particularly useful in children in whom aspirin is not tolerated, either because of gastrointestinal disturbances or because of deafness. In general, ibuprofen has been well tolerated over months and years with occasional rashes as the only side-effect.

2.4 Naproxen

Naproxen suspension has been shown to have the same plasma half-life in children as the tablets in adults (Ansell et al., 1975). Currently, a double-blind study comparing naproxen suspension at a dose of 10mg/kg in two divided doses daily with 80mg/kg of aspirin in 4 divided doses daily is under way. To date, both drugs have been well tolerated and there is little to choose between them with regard to control of pain and stiffness, and the maintenance of function. Tolerance studies are now in progress using the same dosage and despite an occasional complaint about the flavour of the suspension, the naproxen suspension has been well tolerated and side-effects have been minimal. There is considerable parent preference towards twice-daily dosage.

2.5 Flufenamic and Mefenamic Acid

Studies with flufenamic acid have shown it to be reasonably effective as an anti-inflammatory analgesic, but there is a high incidence of diarrhoea and rashes during prolonged therapy. Its use is not recommended. Mefenamic acid in a dosage of 20mg/kg daily in divided doses has proved a useful adjunct in therapy in juvenile chronic polyarthritis (Kent and Ansell, 1975). As has been suggested, its use should be limited to 7 days at any one time because of the possibility of side-effects, such as haemolytic anaemia and steatorrhoea. Its main place is during a period of increased pain in a child already receiving maximum salicylate therapy.

2.6 Tolmetin

A comparative study of children in the USA has shown that 30 to 50mg/kg daily of tolmetin compares favourably with 80 to 100mg/kg per day of aspirin in the control of joint symptoms, during the 3 month comparative study period (Brewer, 1977).

2.7 Phenylbutazone and Oxyphenbutazone

In young children, i.e. below the age of 7 years, side-effects are relatively common. These have included fever, rash, hepatitis and pancytopenia (Gaisford, 1962). The main use of phenylbutazone and oxyphenbutazone would appear to be in that sub-group of children who have a pauci-articular arthritis, usually boys at the age of 9 or 10. This sub-group is related to ankylosing spondylitis as shown by the subsequent development of sacro-iliitis over a few years, or even overt ankylosing spondylitis, often a family history, and usually the presence of HLA B27 antigen (Ansell, 1976). These patients are not easily controlled on high dosages of aspirin, and phenylbutazone, oxyphenbutazone, indomethacin or naproxen may be of more use. The dosage of these drugs should be tailored to the body weight of the patient and it is suggested that something in the order of 5mg/kg daily of phenylbutazone is adequate.

3. Corticosteroid Therapy

This will need to be considered in serious systemic illness, severe joint involvement, particularly associated with deterioration in general health and not responding to the basic regimen already outlined, and in severe chronic iridocyclitis. Because children rapidly show some degree of hypercortisonism with suppression of the hypothalamic pituitary adrenal (HPA) axis, the use of daily corticosteroids in divided doses is undesirable. Once suppressed, the child is at risk for any stressful event, so that a minor episode of diarrhoea and vomiting or other intercurrent infection can precipitate coma. In addition, the majority of children fail to grow and this can be complicated by severe osteoporosis with crush fractures of vertebrae.

For systemic manifestations corticotrophin is useful, and should it need to be continued for a prolonged period, provided the interval between injections is suitably spaced for the type of preparation employed, suppression of the HPA axis does not occur and growth usually continues (Zutshi et al., 1971). In practice the ACTH suspended in gelatin, given either daily or on alternate days, allows recovery between injections (Friedman and Greenwood, 1968) as do corticosteroids given as a single dose on alternate days (Soyka, 1972). However, in severe systemic illness, alternate day corticosteroids take longer to control the disease process than does corticotrophin.

For patients whose main indications are serious joint problems with deterioration in general health there is little to choose between alternate day prednisolone, given at anything from 10 to 20mg as a single dose every 48 hours, and a small dose of corticotrophin (gel), 20 units given every 48 hours. More prolonged-acting preparations, such as tetracosactrin, need very careful use if hypercortisonism is to be avoided, with the weekly dose not exceeding 0.5mg. Needless to say, the type of dose indicated here will not completely control all manifestations but will allow the child to cope with physiotherapy, remobilisation and probably even school. There may well be stiffness on the afternoon of the off day and in the morning that they are due for their steroid preparation. This can usually be overcome by the suitably timed use of a non-steroidal anti-inflammatory analgesic such as indomethacin or a propionic acid derivative such as naproxen or ibuprofen, in addition to their salicylate background therapy.

Once a child has been put on daily divided dose corticosteroid therapy with its associated dangers, it is extremely difficult to return them to once daily, let alone alternate day regimens. Attempts to do this are associated with acute exacerbations of arthritis and often systemic features, while the child may have symptoms of hypoadrenalism on the day off steroid. Because of this, if the child needs to be converted from daily divided doses to alternate day therapy, one usually brings the patient into hospital and starts by changing to a single morning dose. Only when the child has adjusted to the change does one start to reduce the dose on the alternate day. This can be done gradually or suddenly. If the latter, one increases to twice the usual daily dose on 1 day and gives 2mg prednisolone as a single morning dose on the alternate day. This dose of prednisolone needs to be continued until there is evidence that the resting plasma cortisols have risen to normal levels. Prednisolone may then be discontinued without the child becoming generally unwell and apathetic on the alternate day. After even a short period of daily divided doses it may take anything up to 6 or 12 months to transfer a child to a single dose of steroids on alternate days. It is extremely important, however, that this is done if growth is to be resumed, osteoporosis to improve and recovery of the HPA axis to occur (Ansell and Bywaters, 1974).

4. 'Specific' Antirheumatic Drugs

These slow acting, 'long-term' agents which appear to alter the course of the disease include chloroquine, gold and penicillamine (chapter III). The indications for these agents are: (1) severe, persistent activity with functional or radiological deterioration despite good basic management, or (2) to control disease activity in a child already steroid dependent, and thus allow reduction in dosage. It is rarely necessary to consider such drugs in seronegative chronic polyarthritis of childhood of less than 2 years duration, but if activity continues for more than 3 or 4 years they will need to be seriously considered. In those cases in which IgM rheumatoid factor is present they should be considered early, preferably as soon as erosions have been seen to develop. It is important that full supportive therapy is continued until these drugs become effective, which is a minimum of 12 weeks, and only then can non-steroidal anti-inflammatory analgesics be gradually withdrawn. It may be necessary to continue gold and penicillamine for several years to control the disease activity adequately.

4.1 Chloroquine and Hydroxychloroquine

Although these antimalarial agents have been used extensively in Scandinavia, there have been relatively few formal studies on their place in chronic polyarthritis of childhood. In general, we have tended to use them when we have not felt the disease quite severe enough to warrant gold or penicillamine; in cases when these drugs are contraindicated, because of difficulties of regular blood control, or refusal by parents; or when side-effects have occurred with gold or penicillamine.

The dosage should be tailored to the patients weight, and it is suggested that 4mg/kg a day of chloroquine phosphate and between 5 and 7mg/kg a day of hydroxychloroquine (Laaksonon et al., 1974) will prevent the development of serious side-effects. The most important side-effect is corneal deposition, which is suggested by Laaksonon and her colleagues as a sign of overdosage. It is reversible, and on stopping the chloroquine or hydroxychloroquine the depositions are absorbed. The real problem is that occasionally macular degeneration has been seen in antimalarial therapy. Because of this, these drugs should only be used when adequate monitoring of ocular function is available.

At the end of 6 months, if there has been no effect at all, it is desirable to reconsider whether other drugs should be employed. If there has been a considerable improvement, the child shoul be transferred to an alternate day regimen, and attempts made to wean them off the antimalarials gradually so that no more than a maximum

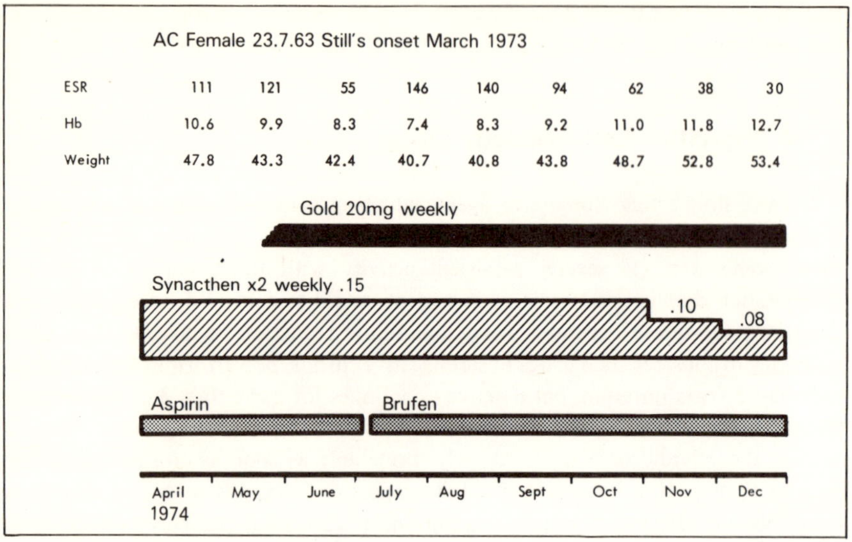

Fig. 1. Gold (sodium aurothiomalate) therapy, showing fall in ESR as well as the ability to reduce synacthen. Note the falling haemoglobin on aspirin, which was associated with positive occult blood. On changing to ibuprofen the haemoglobin rose, continuing to rise as the disease state improved.

of 2 years is given in any 1 course. In addition to the possibility of eye problems, bleaching of the hair is occasionally encountered. As yet, neuromuscular problems have not been recorded in juvenile chronic polyarthritis.

4.2 Gold

Gold, as sodium aurothiomalate, does not appear to be more toxic in children than in adults (chapter III; sect. 1.3). The dosage can either be 1mg/kg body weight given weekly, or standardised at 10mg weekly for children with a body weight of up to 19kg and 20mg weekly for those between 20 and 30kg, increasing to the adult dosage of 50mg weekly. Injections should be given weekly for a minimum period of 6 months unless the side-effects of proteinuria, rash or blood dyscrasias occur. It is only after 6 months that it is possible to appreciate whether therapy is affecting the underlying disease process. It is therefore desirable to have a full appraisal at this time. If there has been no clinical or haematological effect, as judged by a reduction in the number of joints showing soft tissue swelling, a falling ESR and a rising haemoglobin (fig. 1), it may be well worth considering changing to another drug. If there is some benefit, therapy should be continued weekly for a further 6 months unless untoward effects occur. If there is marked benefit, therapy can be reduced to fortnightly, or even monthly; depending on the state of remission of the disease.

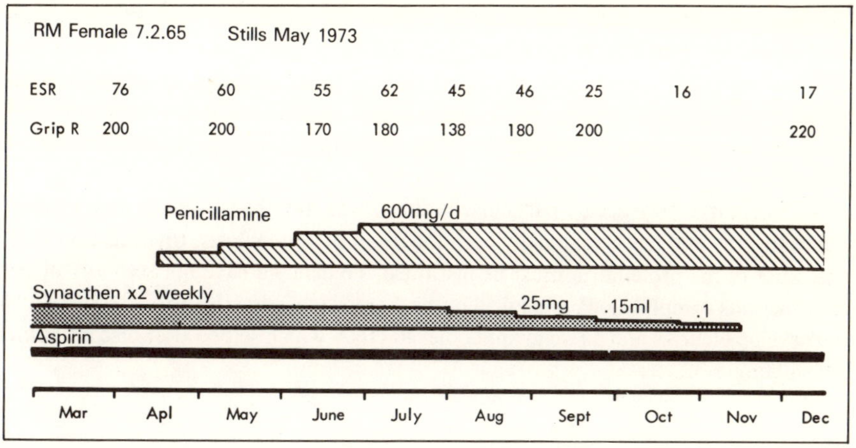

Fig. 2. Penicillamine therapy, showing fall in ESR, improvement in function and withdrawal of tetracosactrin.

At the end of the second 6 month period, the whole situation needs review. If satisfactory improvement has occurred, maintenance therapy of monthly dosage, reducing to 2-monthly, should usually be continued for several years, since there is a significant relapse rate after a single 6 month course of gold (Moller et al., 1969).

The development of persistent proteinuria during gold therapy should lead to investigation for amyloidosis, a much more common cause for persistent proteinuria in juveniles than gold nephropathy, although the latter has been seen on occasions. In our experience, some 60% of children with severe progressive disease can be expected to improve on gold (Moller et al., 1969).

4.3 Penicillamine

Penicillamine has only been used in children for a relatively short period of time. The optimum dosage is stil not certain. Schairer et al. (1976) used 30mg/kg body weight daily, while we have used slowly increasing dosages beginning with 50mg daily in children weighing less than 20kg and 100mg daily in those over 20kg, increasing up to a maximum of 450mg and 600mg daily respectively. We have aimed to maintain this therapy for up to 2 years unless the disease goes into remission, in which case we reduce to a maintenance dosage of 125 or 250mg daily. Comparative studies with gold (Ansell and Hall, 1977) suggest that both drugs are equally effective (fig. 2).

While at present penicillamine poses rather more problems in management, perhaps because of our lack of experience, it is generally preferred by the patient and parents, probably because it is given by mouth rather than by injection and because we have been able to carry out monthly monitoring rather more quickly than with gold injections. Side-effects have been very similar to gold, but it is of interest that children have not complained of disturbance of taste, although anorexia is occasionally noticed. Rash, transient leucopenia and thrombocytopenia have occurred but have not necessarily required stopping of therapy, only some modification of dosage.

Proteinuria may occur, particularly after some months of satisfactory maintenance therapy and has occasionally been the result of amyloidosis. Investigation as to the cause of the proteinuria must be instituted. To date we have not seen any of the more serious complications of penicillamine therapy (chapter III; sect. 2.3) but 1 child did develop pleurisy and a rise in antibodies to DNA which settled after discontinuing penicillamine.

5. Immunosuppressive Therapy

Because of the possible mutagenic and oncogenic effects of these drugs they need to be used with extreme caution. They should certainly not be introduced as a routine in the management of active seronegative chronic polyarthritis of childhood. They will, however, need to be considered if amyloidosis, the one potentially fatal complication of juvenile chronic polyarthritis, is present, or if very serious side-effects have occurred on other forms of therapy.

Azathioprine in a daily dosage of 2.5mg/kg body weight is of use, but blood monitoring is essential as there is a definite risk of suppression of the bone marrow (Kolle, 1969). Azathioprine is less likely to have serious mutagenic effects than alkylating agents such as chlorambucil or cyclophosphamide and is therefore recommended for those cases when immunosuppressive therapy is indicated because of serious side-effects from other drugs. Although there has been one encouraging report on the use of cyclophosphamide (Skogland et al., 1971) another does not support this (Walters, 1972). Cyclophosphamide cannot be recommended because of the possibility of permanent damage to the bladder, and hair loss can be very distressing.

In our hands, the alkylating agent chlorambucil has been particularly effective in controlling disease activity in those children having the complication of amyloidosis and has been found to be acceptable by the patients (Schnitzer and Ansell, 1977). From the haematological point of view it has been difficult to monitor therapy and viral infections, particularly herpes zoster and chicken pox, have been troublesome, often requiring cessation of therapy and the administration of prophylactic gamma globulin. The dosage employed was 0.15mg/kg initially, but this has always had to be tailored to the individual as a result of regular blood monitoring aimed to control disease activity, while maintaining the white blood count above 3000 per cu mm and the platelets above 120,000 per cu mm.

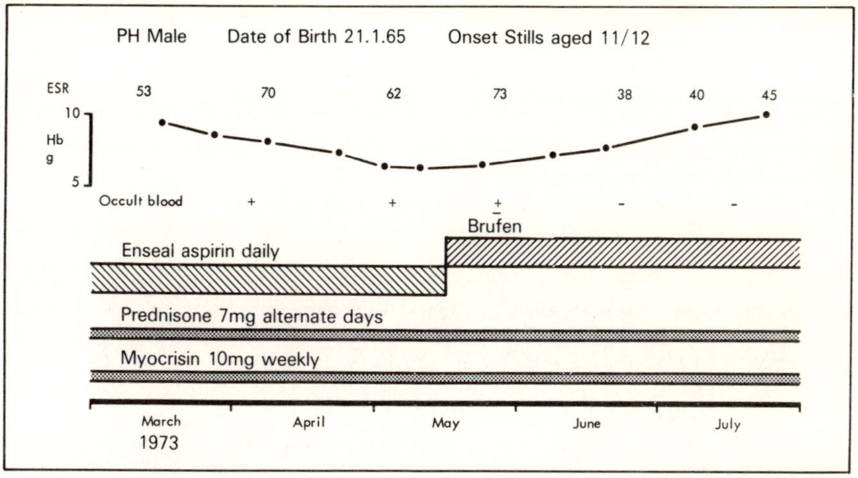

Fig. 3. Combined drug therapy showing the problem of falling haemoglobin with positive occult bloods, which improved after transfer from aspirin to ibuprofen. The alternate day prednisone was at the lowest dosage the child could tolerate and as yet there had been little effect on gold.

6. Combined Drug Therapy

A small proportion of children with juvenile chronic polyarthritis have a prolonged course of severe activity. In such circumstances, it may be necessary to use a number of medications to control the disease process. To avoid side-effects from daily divided dosage of corticosteroids, the patient is put onto an alternate day regimen and non-steroidal anti-inflammatory analgesics given (fig. 3). In the case illustrated, it was necessary to change to ibuprofen because aspirin caused gastrointestinal bleeding, 'specific' antirheumatic drugs are added with the idea of gradually withdrawing the corticosteroids once the disease activity comes under control, but this may take months or years. The same is true for the occasional case when it is desirable to use an immunosuppressive agent. Only when these drugs become effective is it reasonable to attempt to withdraw first corticosteroids and then, considerably later, non-steroidal anti-inflammatory analgesics and finally all antirheumatic therapy.

References and Recommended Reading

Ansell, B.M.: Ibuprofen in the management of Still's disease. Practitioner 211: 659 (1973).

Ansell, Barbara M.: Treatment of juvenile chronic polyarthritis. Clinics in Rheumatic Diseases 1: 443 (1975).

Ansell, B.M.: Differing patterns in juvenile chronic polyarthritis; in Hughes (Ed) Modern Topics in Rheumatology, p.65 (Heinemann, London 1976).

Ansell, B.M. and Bywaters, E.G.L.: Alternate-day corticosteroid therapy in juvenile chronic polyarthritis. Journal of Rheumatology 1: 176 (1974).

Ansell, B.M.and Hall, M.A.: Arthritis and Rheumatism Supplement. In Press (1977).

Ansell, B.M.; Hanna, D.B. and Stoppard, M.: Naprosyn absorption in children. Current Medical Research and Opinion 3: 46 (1975).

Athreya, B.H.: Aspirin induced hepatotoxicity in juvenile rheumatoid arthritis. a prospective study. Arthritis and Rheumatism 18: 347 (1975).

Brewer, E.: Arthritis and Rheumatism Supplement. In Press (1977).

Bywaters, E.G.L.: The management of juvenile chronic polyarthritis. Bulletin of Rheumatic Diseases 27: 882 (1976-1977).

Friedman, M. and Greenwod, F.C.: The effect of prolonged ACTH on corticosteroid therapy in children on growth and on pituitary-adrenal and pituitary function. Memoirs of the Society for Endocrinology 17: 249 (1968).

Gaisford, W.: Fatality after oxyphenbutazone in Still's disease. British Medical Journal 2: 15 (1962).

Jacobs, J.C.: Sudden death in arthritic children receiving large doses of indomethacin. Journal of the American Medical Association 199: 932 (1967).

Kent, P.A. and Ansell, B.M.: Fenemates in the management of juvenile chronic polyarthritis. European Rheumatology Congress, Helsinki. Scandinavian Journal of Rheumatology Suppl. 8: Abstract 1108 (1975).

Kolle, G.: Knochemarksschadigung bei immunsuppressiver therapie der juvenilen rheumatoiden arthritis und des Still sydnrome mit Azathioprin. Deutsche medizinische Wochenschrift 94: 2268 (1969).

Laaksonen, A.L.; Koskiahde, V. and Juva, K.: Dosage of antimalarial drugs for children with juvenile rheumatoid arthritis and systemic lupus erythematosus. A clinical study with determination of serum concentrations of chloroquine and hydroxychloroquine. Scandinavian Journal of Rheumatology 3: 103 (1974).

Makela, A.L.: Dosage of salicylates for children with juvenile rheumatoid arthritis. A preliminary report. Scandinavian Journal of Rheumatology 4: 250 (1975).

Moller, P.W.; Ansell, B.M. and Bywaters, E.G.L.: Myocrisin therapy in Still's disease. Proceedings of the 12th International Congress of Rheumatic Diseases, Prague, Abstract No. 675 (1969).

Powell, R.H.: Benorylate in the management of Still's disease. British Medical Journal 1: 145 (1974).

Rich, R. and Johnson, J.: Salicylate hepatotoxicity in patients with juvenile rheumatoid arthritis. Arthritis and Rheumatisim 16: 1 (1973).

Russell, A.S.; Sturge, R.A. and Smith, M.A.: Serum transaminase levels during salicylate therapy. British Medical Journal 2: 428 (1971).

Schairer, H.; Stoeben, E. and Koelle, G.: Preliminary results of a controlled trial of gold salts and penicillamine in treatment of juvenile rheumatoid arthritis. Zeitschrift fur Rheumaforschung 35 (Suppl. 4): 54 (1976).

Schnitzer, T.L. and Ansell, B.M.: Arthritis and Rheumatism supplement. In Press (1977).

Skoglund, R.R.; Schanberger, J.E. and Kaplan, J.M.: Cyclophosphamide therapy for severe juvenile rheumatoid arthritis. American Journal of Diseases of Children 121: 531 (1971).

Soyka, L.F.: Alternate-day corticosteroid therapy. Advances in Pediatrics 19: 47 (1972).

Walters, D.: Poor response in two cases of juvenile rheumatoid arthritis to treatment with cyclophosphamides. Medical Journal of Australia 2: 1070 (1972).

Zutshi, D.W.; Friedman, M. and Ansell, B.M.: Corticotrophin therapy in juvenile chronic polyarthritis (Still's disease) and effect of growth. Archives of Diseases in Childhood 46: 584 (1971).

Chapter XX

Less Common Arthropathies

There are many different types of arthritis. Indeed, about 180 different rheumatological diagnoses can be made (Huskisson and Hart, 1975). Unfortunately for the patients who have them, but fortunately for the doctors who have to remember how to treat them, most have no specific therapy. Reliance must therefore be made on non-specific or symptomatic therapy, as discussed in chapter I; (sect. 3).

1. Miscellaneous Arthropathies

Most of these conditions are benign, and some are self-limiting, so that a policy of using the safest and best-tolerated drugs first is particularly applicable. Conditions which fall into this category include Reiter's disease, yersinia arthritis and other types of reactive or postinfective arthritis, pyrophosphate arthropathy, enteropathic synovitis, Bechet's disease, and the arthritis associated with erythema nodosum and sarcoidosis. Many patients will do well on propionic acid derivatives (chapter II; sect. 5-8) and as in other conditions, the clinician must remember to be prepared to try several to find the best drug for each individual patient.

Patients with more active inflammation; for example, acute cases of Reiter's disease or pyrophosphate arthropathy, may require the more potent anti-inflammatory effect of drugs like indomethacin. Occasionally, in conditions which are self-limiting and when other non-steroidal anti-inflammatory drugs have failed, systemic corticosteroid therapy may be considered, but the dangers of prolonged high dose therapy must always be weighed against the possible benefits (chapt. IV). Intra-articular corticosteroids (chapter V) are certainly useful; for example in acute Reiter's disease or pyrophosphate arthropathy.

2. Arthritis Associated with Malignancy

In some conditions, the availability of non-specific therapy is actually dangerous. One must always remember that some types of arthritis are associated with serious underlying conditions such as malignant disease. Prolonged treatment with non-specific therapy may alleviate the symptoms while the underlying condition progresses. There are many ways in which malignant disease may cause arthritis, including pseudohypertrophic osteoarthropathy, dermatomyositis, referred pain and deposits adjacent to joints. The correct treatment is management of the underlying malignancy.

Myeloma is a condition which most commonly presents as bone or joint pain. Specific therapy with courses of melphalan and prednisolone, or other combinations of cytotoxic drugs provide the best means of controlling the disease although additional symptomatic therapy may be required. The same applies to other malignant diseases complicated by arthritis.

3. Familial Meditteranean Fever

This is a condition characterised by attacks of arthritis, fever and serositis. The treatment of the condition has been totally changed by the finding that colchicine in a dose of 0.5mg 2 or 3 times daily prevents attacks in most patients (Editorial, 1975).

4. Paget's Disease

Paget's disease is another condition for which specific therapy is now available. The disease is common in elderly people and causes bone and joint pain. Many patients can be managed with analgesic and anti-inflammatory drugs, but some have intractable pain, when specific therapy should be considered. There are three different approaches: mithramycin, calcitonin and disodium etidronate (EHDP).

Mithramycin is a cytotoxic drug which may inhibit osteoblasts and thereby new bone formation. It is given in a dose of 15mg/kg body weight daily for 10 days by intravenous infusion over 6 hours in a solution of 5% dextrose. Serum calcium and liver function tests should be monitored daily. There are few side-effects, but nausea, abnormal liver function tests and hypocalcaemia may occur. Pain is often relieved within a few days of starting treatment; most patients respond and recurrence is unusual at least over the first 5 years (Russell and Lentle, 1974). Biochemical abnormalities of the disease, such as raised alkaline phosphatase and increased hydroxyproline excretion, improve slowly.

EHDP is diphosphonate which is believed to act by inhibiting the formation of hydroxyapatite crystals in bone. It is given in a dose of up to 20mg/kg EHDP a day, by mouth. Absorption is poor and, although the drug is cleared from the plasma within 24 hours of a single dose, it accumulates in bone and is only slowly removed. About 80% of patients with Paget's disease show substantial improvement in biochemical parameters of the disease, but only about 50% show substantial clinical improvement (Russell et al., 1974). Nausea and diarrhoea occur occasionally, raised serum phosphate levels are common and there may be a slight increase in the incidence of fractures with prolonged high-dose treatment. Treatment should not normally be continued for longer than 6 months but further courses can be given to treat recurrence of pain.

Calcitonin inhibits osteoclastic activity in bone and reduces bone turnover. Two preparations are available. Synthetic salmon calcitonin is given in a dose of 100 international units daily for 3 to 6 months then at a maintenance dose of 50 units 3 times weekly. Extracted porcine calcitonin is given in a dose of 160 international units daily for 3 to 6 months, then 80 units 3 times weekly. Both are given by intramuscular injection. Pain relief is achieved in about one-third of all patients, although biochemical improvement is usual. Calcitonin begins to exert its effect within 2 to 6 weeks of the start of treatment so that if it hasn't worked after 6 weeks, it won't. If it achieves a response, treatment should be continued for a year, then stopped and a further course given in the event of recurrence. Side-effects include anorexia and nausea. Since allergic reactions may occur, it is wise to give a test dose of intradermal calcitonin initially.

5. Other Conditions

Palindromic rheumatism is probably in most cases a variant of rheumatoid arthritis in which there are attacks of arthritis which resolve spontaneously. Anti-inflammatory therapy with indomethacin for example, may be useful during the attack but for patients with frequent severe attacks, penicillamine should be considered. A dose of 250mg daily seems to stop the attacks in many cases (Huskisson, 1976).

Psychogenic rheumatism describes the occurrence of joint pains in patients with psychological disturbances, of which the most common are anxiety and depression. The use of antianxiety drugs such as diazepam in the former and antidepressants such as imipramine in the latter is useful. It is pointless to give analgesics, which don't work.

In the so-called reflex dystrophies, *shoulder hand syndrome and neuralgic amytrophy,* intramuscular ACTH is often strikingly effective. It should be given in an initial dose of 40 units on alternate days, reducing to the lowest possible dose. Corticosteroid therapy, with oral prednisolone, is also required in *chronic active hepatitis,* a condition in which joint pain is not uncommon.

Arthritis is the major manifestation of *haemophilia* and chronic changes in joints used to be one of the major problems of this disease. The use of factor VIII in this disease, and factor IX in *Christmas disease*, can prevent bleeding episodes and early treatment is essential when they occur.

Other conditions which may present with arthritis but which require specific therapy include *hypothyroidism*. Replacement doses of thyroxine produce gradual improvement in the arthritis which is not usually helped by anti-inflammatory drugs and may be made worse by phenylbutazone, which occasionally produces subthyroidism and goitre in normal patients. Vitamin D is required for *osteomalacia and rickets* which may present with pain in the joints. In *Whipples disease*, there is evidence of an infective agent in the small intestine and treatment with tetracycline is effective.

There are some unusual infections which cause arthritis and require particular antimicrobial agents. In *leprosy*, clofazimine may be useful to control the reactions and dapsone is required to eradicate the disease. Tuberculosis, brucellosis, mycoplasma, lymphogranuloma venereum, helminths and fungi can all cause arthritis and require appropriate antimicrobial agent directed at the particular causative organism.

References and Recommended Reading

Editorial: Colchicine in familial Mediterranean fever. British Medical Journal 3: 60 (1975).

Huskisson, E.C.: Treatment of palindromic rheumatism with D-penicillamine. British Medical Journal 2: 979 (1976).

Huskisson, E.C. and Hart, F.D.: Joint Disease: All the Arthropathies, 2nd Ed (John Wright, Bristol 1975).

Russell, A.S. and Lentle, B.C.: Mithramycin therapy in Paget's disease. Canadian Medical Association Journal 110: 397 (1974).

Russell, R.G.G.; Smith, R.; Preston, C.; Walton, A.J. and Wood, C.G.: Diphosphonates in Paget's disease. Lancet 1: 894 (1974).

Chapter XXI

Adjunctive Drug Therapy in Arthritis

A variety of other drugs can be used to relieve anxiety or depression, improve disturbed sleep patterns, or improve general well-being.

1. Anaemia

Anaemia can occur in patients suffering from a variety of forms of arthritis, sometimes from the disease itself, sometimes from the therapy given, sometimes from chance and coincidence. Mowat (1971, 1972) observed that a moderate hypochromic normocytic anaemia is a common feature of rheumatoid arthritis; microcytosis being uncommon and hypochromia appearing before microcytosis, the opposite of what is seen in iron deficiency anaemia. With active disease the plasma iron is low: the haemoglobin concentration and plasma iron levels can be correlated with the erythrocyte sedimentation rate and disease activity.

In rheumatoid arthritis absorption of iron is normal or reduced, but in the presence of anaemia and a low plasma iron, absorption is usually increased. Mowat observes that the hypochromic, normocytic anaemia in patients with rheumatoid arthritis rarely responds to oral iron but that intramuscular doses of iron sorbitol (iron sorbitol citric acid complex) or intramuscular or intravenous iron dextran will increase haemoglobin concentrations in most patients. If intravenous iron dextran is used, an initial test dose must be given. Reactions by this route are common and include fever, constitutional upset and occasionally exacerbations of the rheumatoid arthritis, probably a hypersensitivity reaction to dextran (Reddy and Lewis, 1969; Lloyd and Williams, 1970). The failure of oral iron to increase the haemoglobin levels in most patients is unlikely to be due to the mild degree of malabsorption from the gastrointestinal tract, but probably reflects a failure to overcome the avidity of the reticuloendothelial system for iron, only the larger amounts given to the plasma by parenteral therapy being likely to reach the bone marrow.

The treatment of the anaemia is essentially the treatment of the rheumatoid arthritis: agents, such as corticosteroids or corticotrophin, which reduce the activity of the disease, will improve the anaemia. Whittingham et al. (1967) and Mowat et al. (1969) found that the plasma iron values could be restored to normal within 72 hours by such therapy and the latter group of workers found a mean rise of 2.05g/100ml (358µmol/L) over a 2 week period.

When there is evidence of iron folate or vitamin B_{12} deficiency, however, the treatment is obviously to replace the deficit. Megaloblastic anaemia, when it occurs in rheumatoid arthritis, is more likely to be due to folate than to vitamin B_{12} deficiency. Secondary sideroblastic anaemia occurs very rarely in rheumatoid arthritis and deficiency of pyridoxine and/or folate are important causal factors (MacGibbon and Mollin, 1965). What has been said of the anaemia in rheumatoid arthritis applies to a lesser degree to other inflammatory arthropathies and to polymyalgia arteritica, but the anaemia in systemic lupus erythematosus is often haemolytic, responding usually to corticosteroid therapy unless uraemia is present (Dubois, 1974).

2. Anaemia Due to Therapy

Anaemia in any of the rheumatic disorders may be complicated by or entirely due to the therapy given. Any of the anti-inflammatory drugs from corticosteroids and aspirin to ibuprofen may occasionally cause gastrointestinal bleeding with secondary anaemia, sometimes sudden and prostrating. Aplastic anaemia may result from phenylbutazone, oxyphenbutazone, gold or a cytotoxic (immunosuppressive) agent. Fatal results are often precipitated in such cases by haemorrhage resulting from platelet deficiency.

3. Vitamin Deficiencies

Low vitamin levels in the diet of patients with arthritis may occasionally, though rarely in developed countries, play a part in causing symptoms.

In rheumatoid arthritis, blood levels of vitamin C may be low (Forster and Engleman, 1961), but there is little or no evidence that administration of ascorbic acid improves therapeutic results, unless the patient is already scorbutic or sub-scorbutic, as may occur in crippled patients living alone with inadequate nutrition, food faddists or chronic alcoholics.

Thiamine and co-carboxylase levels may also be decreased in the serum (Kodama, 1959). It is unlikely to be of importance in arthritic patients, unless diet is grossly deficient, the patient is an alcoholic or has a chronic mental illness or a severe chronic gastrointestinal disorder.

Kalliomaki et al. (1960) found riboflavine blood levels reduced in rheumatoid arthritis. Angular stomatitis may rapidly respond to large doses of the vitamin, but often does not, as, according to Davidson and Wright (1972) a common cause is not riboflavine-deficiency, but ill-fitting dentures associated with candidiasis.

Nicotinic acid blood levels, according to Kalliomaki et al. (1960) in Finland, are also occasionally depressed in rheumatoid arthritis. McKusick et al. (1964) found pyridoxine excretion to be diminished significantly in rheumatoid arthritis, but any practical significance of either of these findings is unclear.

4. Anxiety

Antianxiety drugs are of modest use in the arthritic and rheumatic disorders, but they do play a part in quietening the agitated patient and diminishing her anxiety in some cases. 30 years ago, phenobarbitone and amylobarbitone (amobarbital) in small doses were the stand-by, but the benzodiazepine compounds, diazepam and chlordiazepoxide, have very largely replaced them as useful and effective agents; very much less liable to produce drug interactions, adverse effects and abuse. Many patients find the benzodiazepines, diazepam in particular, too sedating, but others improve not only psychologically but physically also. There is considerable individual tolerance, particularly with diazepam, when 1 patient will do well on 10mg 3 times daily another will become sleepy on 2mg 3 times daily.

It is as well for the clinician treating anxious patients to appreciate that in some cases drugs may precipitate or aggravate their symptoms. Almost any of the sympathomimetic amines can produce anxiety-like symptoms, and even sedative drugs given for anxiety may sometimes aggravate the condition they were intended to help. Adequate reassurance often removes the need for antianxiety drugs which may harm the patient in some cases by reducing his fighting spirit, in others by causing drug dependence or abuse. In this respect the barbiturates are best avoided. Any muscle relaxation diazepam causes in the arthritic disorders is mostly if not entirely through its central actions. The claim that diazepam has antirheumatic properties remains non-proven.

5. Depression

Depression is common in chronic sufferers with rheumatic disease. It may be primary (endogenous) and only aggravated by the arthritic condition, but in many cases is a by-product of the chronic frustrating and painful disease. It is of primary importance to give the patient time to talk and discuss her condition ('complaining time') with her clinician, physiotherapist, nurse or occupational therapist. Antidepressant drugs, although helpful, should be used with considerable discrimination only after adequate psychiatric assessment by her clinician and, in selected cases, her psychiatrist.

Some tricyclic antidepressants such as amitriptyline, trimipramine and doxepin have a marked sedative action, imipramine less so, while others such as protriptyline have little or none. The antianxiety or sedative effect of the tricyclics occurs earlier than the antidepressant or 'mood elevating' effect. The particular antidepressant, when and if the time comes to use it, should be selected with these facts in mind. Tricyclics should be given in full dosage (e.g. 75 to 150mg amitriptyline daily), with smaller dosage in the elderly. A single daily dose of a sedative compound at bedtime is convenient to the patient and also benefits disturbed sleep patterns (see section 6). Although it has been said that endogenous depression responds better to the tricyclic antidepressants and exogenous or reactive depression to the monoamine oxidase (MAO) inhibitors, this is not always so. Because of the wide range of drug and food interactions with the MAOIs, the tricyclics are usually the drug of first choice. If the MAO inhibitors or electroconvulsive therapy are to be used, the patient should be treated in a psychiatric unit.

It must be emphasised that the large majority of depressed patients will recover eventually without treatment, but in the meantime their arthritic symptoms may worsen even if the physical signs remain unchanged. Depression left untreated induces a negative response to life which may extend to the action of the patient's antirheumatic drug therapy, which may become less effective in controlling symptoms. The addition of antidepressants to the antirheumatic programme of drug therapy may sometimes improve the patient's symptoms considerably.

6. Insomnia

The main factor preventing normal sleep in most patients with active arthritis is pain, but insomnia as such may play a part. Insomnia + pain + anxiety and depression is an 'ugly' mixture and many rheumatoids, spondylitics and other sufferers are often at their worst at night. Heavy sedation is, however, to be avoided where active inflammatory disease is present as it often makes the waking and rising in the morning in conditions such as rheumatoid arthritis or ankylosing spondylitis, considerably worse. Sedation should therefore be not unduly heavy and given with appropriate anti-inflammatory and/or analgesic agents.

The most appropriate hypnotics, taken shortly before retiring, are nitrazepam (5 to 10mg), flurazepam (15 to 30mg), diazepam (5 to 10mg). Generally speaking, smaller doses (i.e. half) are preferred in the elderly: there is a greater tendency to confusion on rising in the night and a greater tendency to postural hypotension. The extremities are weaker and fractures happen more readily in the aged osteoporotic sufferers. Triclofos (1g) and dichloralphenazone (650 to 130mg) are usually well tolerated by the elderly, but, as in most therapeutic situations, there is great individual variability and tolerance. Where depression is a feature, tricyclic antidepressants with a sedative action such as amitriptyline, trimipramine or doxepin, given on retiring, are to be preferred. Their use may eliminate the need for hypnotics.

References and Recommended Reading

Davidson, S. and Wright, T.J.: in Davidson and MacLeod (Eds) The Principles and Practice of Medicine. 10th ed, p.189 (Churchill Livingstone, Edinburgh 1972).

Dubois, E.L.: Lupus Erythematosus, 2nd ed, p.165 (University of Southern California Press, Los Angeles 1974).

Forster, J.E. and Engleman, E.P.: The effect of adrenal corticosteroid therapy on blood ascorbic acid levels in rheumatoid arthritis. Arthritis and Rheumatism 4: 418 (1961).

Kalliomaki, J.L.; Laine, V.A.I. and Markkanen, T.K.: Urinary excretion of thiamine, riboflavine, nicotinic acid, and pantothenic acid in patients with rheumatoid arthritis. Acta Medica Scandinavica 166: 275 (1960).

Kodama, T.: Acta Medica Okayama 13: 137 (1959); cited in Hollander and McCarty (Eds) Arthritis, 8th Ed, p.380 (Lea & Febiger, Philadelphia 1972).

Lloyd, K.N. and Williams, P.: Reactions to total dose infusion of iron dextran in rheumatoid arthritis. British Medical Journal 2: 323 (1970).

MacGibbon, B.H. and Mollin, D.L.: Sideroblastic anaemia in man: observations on seventy cases. British Journal of Haematology 11: 59 (1965).

McKusick, A.B.; Sherwin, R.W.; Jones, L.G. and Hsu, J.M.: Urinary excretion of pyridoxine and 4-pyridoxic acid in rheumatoid arthritis. Arthritis and Rheumatism 7: 636 (1974).

Mowat, A.G.: in Hill (Ed) Modern Trends in Rheumatology, Vol. 2, p.106 (Butterworths London 1971).

Mowat, A.G.: Haematologic abnormalities in rheumatoid arthritis. Seminars in Arthritis and Rheumatism 1: 195 (1972).

Mowat, A.G.; Hothershall, T.E. and Aitchison, W.R.C.: Nature of anaemia in rheumatoid arthritis. XI. Changes in iron metabolism induced by the administration of corticotrophin. Annals of the Rheumatic Diseases 28: 303 (1969).

Reddy, P.S. and Lewis, M.: The adverse effect of intravenous iron-dextran in rheumatoid arthritis. Arthritis and Rheumatism 12: 454 (1969).

Whittingham, S.F.; Balazs, N.D.H. and Mackay, I.R.: Effect of corticosteroids on serum iron levels in SLE and rheumatoid arthritis. Medical Journal of Australia 2: 639 (1967).

Subject Index

B

C

D

N

O

P

R

S